SEXY
FOREVER

THREE RIVERS PRESS

NEW YORK

SEXY FOREVER

How to Fight Fat After Forty

SUZANNE SOMERS

Copyright © 2010 by Suzanne Somers

All rights reserved.
Published in the United States by Three Rivers Press,
an imprint of the Crown Publishing Group,
a division of Random House, Inc., New York.
www.crownpublishing.com

Three Rivers Press and the Tugboat design are registered trademarks
of Random House, Inc.

Originally published in hardcover in the United States
by Crown Archetype, an imprint of the Crown Publishing Group,
a division of Random House, Inc., New York, in 2010.

Library of Congress Cataloging-in-Publication Data
is available upon request.

ISBN 978-0-307-58852-4
eISBN 978-0-307-58853-1

Printed in the United States of America

Book design by Diane Hobbing of Snap-Haus Graphics
Cover design by Caroline Somers and Danielle Shapero-Rudolph
Cover photography by Cindy Gold

10 9 8 7 6 5 4 3 2 1

First Paperback Edition

For Alan, always

Illnesses do not come upon us out of the blue. They are developed from small daily sins against nature. When enough sins have accumulated, illnesses will suddenly appear.

—*Hippocrates*

ACKNOWLEDGMENTS

There are three women, so valuable to the completion of this book, it's difficult to know in what order to give them their due praise: Caroline Somers, Heather Jackson, and Marsha Yanchuck.

Caroline Somers is my daughter-in-law, my business partner, protector of the brand, and mother of my granddaughters. When Caroline takes on an assignment, she approaches it with an excellence and tenacity that boggles the mind. She labored over the program sections, testing recipes in her personal kitchen, and was sending me e-mails after completion often at three a.m. She cares, she does her job perfectly, and without her I would not have made my deadline. I love her and am extremely grateful to have her in my life for every reason I can think of.

Heather Jackson, editor extraordinaire; this is our third book together and each project becomes easier and silkier under her steady but firm guidance. She has a wonderful soul, a kind heart, and a great brain. Her organizational skills are extraordinary, and I depend on her to pull each book out of me.

Marsha Yanchuck, who I have worked with for over three decades . . . to whom I literally turn over the resource section of my books, as I did with this one. Because of Marsha, the reader can access information, whether it be from the back of the book or from references on my website. Marsha has set it up so that doctors in many cities, states, and countries are easily found, a service I know is appreciated by not only myself but my readers. And that she is my grammar and spelling police is no small thing. Thank you.

Brenda Watson, the foremost authority on gut health in America and possibly the world, was invaluable in teaching me and coaching me on the complexities of the gut as it pertains to weight loss. Spending so much time learning with her was akin to getting my master's. In the process, she uncovered food intolerances and allergies plaguing not only myself but members of my family.

Dr. Jonathan Wright, the father of bioidentical hormone treatment in America, who once again so generously gave me his time and knowledge to connect the dots regarding hormonal imbalance and weight gain. His downhome way of explaining and breaking down the hormonal system and its effects is endlessly fascinating to me. He is a national treasure and deeply appreciated.

Dr. Nick Gonzalez, who is always there on the other end of the telephone or on e-mail with his profound command and knowledge of what makes the body sick and how to bring it back to balance.

Bill Faloon, editor of *Life Extension* magazine, along with Dr. Scott Fogle and Peter Zhang, M.D., Ph.D., all part of the extraordinary LE scientific advisory board, who once again took on the tedious task of going over this book, page by page, to correct it for accuracy and integrity. When readers take learning so seriously from my books, knowing that I am scientifically and factually correct, due to obtaining the stamp of approval from these informed men, gives me great peace of mind.

A big thank-you to my nutritionist, Cristiana Paul, M.S., who always brings so much to my books.

The girls in my office, my dear and valuable assistants Julie Turkel and Jordyn Goodman; they keep my life running and make it possible by taking care of everything, allowing for room in my head to put out these books. They are joyous girls and totally professional. I love working with both of them and appreciate them deeply.

Thank you to Linda Chae for her expertise on toxicity and the skin, and thank you to all the authors listed at the back of this book for the information I garnered while doing research for this book.

My team at Crown; I have lost count of how many books we have done together, all I know is this is my twentieth book, most of them done with Crown and most of them bestsellers. What an incredible ride we've been on together. Thanks to dear Tina Constable, Maya Mavjee, Philip Patrick,

Jill Flaxman, Annsley Rosner, and Patty Berg. Thanks to the production team: production editor Christine Tanigawa, production manager Luisa Francavilla, in-house designer Songhee Kim, and freelance designer Diane Hobbing of Snap-Haus Graphics.

And big thanks to my new friends at Everyday Health: Mike Keriakos who has been after me to use the word *sexy* in combination with weight loss in a book for the past five years; darling Steven Petrow; Vince Errico, Sarah Hutter, Debbie Strong, Hilary Hayward, Maureen MacDonald, and Alice Calista Cronin.

Many thanks to the design team for the beautiful jacket. Under the creative direction of Caroline Somers, Danielle Shapero has been the graphic designer for my brand for the past decade. Danielle, I can always count on you to keep it fresh, clean, and beautiful. And special thanks to Mark Wilkinson for the ominous back jacket panel of toxins. And to Laura Duffy, the designer at Crown, for helping us stay in the margins and get it all just right! Special thanks to my amazing photographer, Cindy Gold, and her ace team, Paul Craig, John Guarente, and Bonnie Holland, for another great cover shot.

Thank you to my friend and doctor Michael Galitzer, for his beautiful foreword and for always reminding me it's mind, body, and spirit.

Thank you to my attorney Marc Chamlin for another book together. And a big thank you to my literary agent David Vigliano who pushed for this project for three years. Good idea, David.

Thank you to Shirani and Farook, who make my life so comfortable, for Shirani's great soup every afternoon giving me sustenance followed by the bowl of fresh fruit cut into bite-size pieces. Thanks to my very savvy, very sexy publicist, Sandi Mendelson. Thank you, Dave Henson, I couldn't write my books without your computer help.

And last but not least, my husband, Alan Hamel, whom I love deeply and who makes it all happen.

CONTENTS

CONTENTS

FOREWORD

God bless Suzanne Somers. I have had the honor of knowing and working with her for the past six years. Suzanne is a health guru. She is a health hero who has single-handedly had an enormous impact on improving the health of our society. In her books, she has presented scientifically based, cutting-edge information through her interviews with esteemed physicians. *The Sexy Years* showed women that they did not have to suffer with the symptoms of menopause and could improve their health by taking bioidentical hormones. In *Ageless*, Suzanne led us into the world of antiaging medicine, where anyone can optimize their health through the proper use of optimal nutrition, dietary supplements, exercise, bioidentical hormones, and stress reduction. *Breakthrough* continued the antiaging theme and showed us how future technologies such as stem cells and nanotechnology will lead to even greater levels of health. And then there was *Knockout*, a wonderful book that empowers and gives hope to all of us who either seek to prevent cancer or are looking for new strategies to defeat it. These four outstanding books provided us with the tools needed to prevent serious illness, and optimize health and longevity.

In this book, *Sexy Forever*, Suzanne states that the best way to lose weight is to get healthy. She perfectly describes the environmental threats to our health while giving us a road map of what to do and what not to do. So how does one get healthy? Here are some of Suzanne's necessary steps for healthy weight loss:

1. Reduce your stress levels.

2. Get at least seven to eight hours of sleep per night.

3. Correct nutrient deficiencies so as to eliminate food cravings.

4. Identify food allergies, especially to gluten and dairy.

5. Improve the health of the gastrointestinal tract.

6. Avoid exposure to toxic chemicals in the air, food, water, and cosmetics.

7. Learn how to effectively lower the toxin load in your body.

8. Exercise in order to create fat burning and increase your basal metabolic rate.

9. Determine your hormone levels and have those levels optimized by seeing a qualified physician experienced in using bioidentical hormones.

10. Avoid insulin resistance by reducing your intake of junk food and simple carbohydrates, while combining exercise with healthy nutritional supplements.

11. Change your beliefs about what is possible.

So how do we change our beliefs about losing weight?

> Most of us continue to look to the past to define possibilities for the future. We go back to a frame of reference in which we were unable to lose weight, and we project that into the present. A belief is nothing more than a feeling of certainty about something. We all had beliefs about the world when we were younger that no longer serve us.

I remember being a kid and thinking that thirty was old!

The first key is to change the beliefs that no longer serve you. The best way is to start developing new attitudes and experiences that cause you to question your old beliefs. The new attitude that you need to adopt is "I will get healthy, and then I will easily be able to lose weight. I know that health equals energy, and the more energy I have, the easier it will be to lose weight."

So how do we get healthy? We must first realize that health is our natural state of being. Disease and illness are but shadows on the river of health. Our bodies are Ferraris that need high-octane fuel. We must feed them organic food. We must limit our exposure to toxins in our environment, and more important, stimulate the elimination systems of the body—the liver, kidneys, and lymph system—to get rid of these toxins that eventually accumulate in our fat. As more and more toxins accumulate in our system, they place severe stress on these organs of elimination. With continued accumulation, the liver, kidneys, and lymph system become less efficient in their ability to excrete these waste products, causing toxins to build first in the connective tissues of the body and then in the organs. The body initially tries to compensate by having the endocrine glands secrete hormones to help stimulate detoxification. Over time these glands become "tired." The end result is an inefficient elimination system with toxin accumulation, coupled with reduced organ and hormonal function—which creates the environment for weight gain.

Suzanne wants us to optimize our hormones in order to become healthy and lose weight. The hormonal system is what most correlates to the emotional person. It is clear that the hormonal system responds to our outlook on the world. Thoughts that make us happy make us well.

Stress is a factor not only in disease but also in the inability to lose weight. There are three main causes of chronic stress. First, we have long-term unhealthy beliefs that cause us to perceive life events as "dangers" and thus trigger an alarm response. Second, we are persistently deprived of the bonding or closeness that all human beings need. Last, we do not get enough of our psychological needs met in our daily environments. These needs are unique to our specific personality type. Some of us need to have fun and excitement; others need acknowledgment of our values; yet others need acknowledgment of our ability to think clearly and logically. Some people need solitude, while some of us need our senses to be richly stimulated.

Please remember the essential theme of Suzanne's book: we first have to improve our health before we can lose weight. The general state of our health is directly related to our consciousness. A change in our health, either for better or for worse, involves a change in our consciousness. Our bodies are constantly renewing themselves. Our consciousness and beliefs can affect the regeneration of cells and organs positively or negatively.

A change in consciousness always involves a change in focus. What excites you, and what are you grateful for? Don't we all want to jump out of bed every morning with a lust and love for life? I bet Suzanne does. See yourself as healthy, and know that this healthy state of being is your natural state.

Health is much, much more than the absence of disease. Health is energy, vitality, passion. Healthy people have physical energy, emotional balance, and spiritual awareness, and simultaneously vibrate on all three levels. Suzanne Somers speaks to all of us in the important work that she is doing in the areas of health, nutrition, and antiaging medicine. She speaks to us as a friend we can trust, believe, and have fun with as we reshape our thoughts and beliefs along with our bodies. *Sexy Forever* is much more than a weight loss book. It gives us the tools to slow the aging process and accelerate the regeneration of the body's cells and tissues. Suzanne Somers has written another great book!

To your health,

Michael Galitzer, M.D.

WHY THIS BOOK?
WHY NOW?

I know just what you are hoping for as you crack open this book. You are hoping for an easy weight loss solution to restore your once beautiful body to its original glory. You are hoping you won't have to give up too many of your favorite foods because you really love to eat. You know you'll have to do some exercise, but you don't have a lot of time, so you hope it won't take too long or make you sweat too much. You are hoping there's no cabbage soup involved. In fact, you'd prefer a magic pill or weight loss powder that will take away your cravings and peel away those pounds—but you don't want it to be dangerous to your health or make you feel jittery like those scary diet pills. You are hoping there is some secret that has been eluding you, since every weight loss program has inevitably failed you in the long run. And you are hoping the knowledge you'll gain about all of the above will make you slim, vibrant, healthy, and absolutely sexy . . . forever.

On this very first page, I can promise you all of that. Within the pages of *Sexy Forever* you will discover

- An easy-to-follow weight loss program filled with rich, delicious foods.

- A moderate exercise program to keep you fit and healthy.

- *Amazing* supplements and weight loss products to catapult you to success. (I can't say *miracle* because the governing bodies get all up in arms about that word!)

- The solution to sleeping eight hours nightly, without drugs, in order to lose weight.

- The key to a healthy digestive tract plus a simple allergy/intolerance test to unlock the hidden secret to your personal food demons that could silently be keeping you overweight or possibly chronically ill.

- Natural hormonal balance—the missing ingredient for every person over forty that *must* be added to make any plan successful. (I have a thing or two to say about this topic!)

- And most important, the unveiling of the thousands of FDA-approved chemicals and toxins surrounding us every day, sabotaging our health and weight—and how to conquer those enemies.

That's quite a promise, I know. I intend to keep it to each and every one of you. Your goal is achievable. I am certain of it, but you must *stay with me* on this journey as we unlock the secrets to what is making us fat in this second half of life. What you will read in these pages may be overwhelming at times. It's not just about fat grams, calories, carbohydrates, or training sessions. The information you are about to digest is actually disturbing. It's so disturbing you may want to close the book and forget everything you've read because what you learn may taint the way you look at a shiny red apple, a perfectly marbled steak, your sparkling clean counter, your favorite scented lotion, your comfortable bed, your gentle baby shampoo, or even your fresh-smelling laundry. *Stay with me.* The information here is your ticket to health and permanent weight loss.

What has happened to us at this age? For women, maybe some of us have just "let ourselves go." Maybe we gained a little weight after the baby was born, got too busy caring for others, and just never got back into shape. For men, maybe we stopped working out and got a little too familiar with fast food, bags of chips, and beer. But what about those of us who try to eat healthy; *really try,* and still don't see any results? I know who you are, and I know you're not eating—at least not very much. I also know you're not very satisfied. In fact, you are probably consuming less food than ever before and most likely your daily fare is predominantly salads. Right?

You're also exercising aren't you? Yoga, Pilates, running, those Curves classes. It all helps . . . well, a little. And, of course, you know it's good for you but, darn, your energy isn't what it used to be. You really aren't feeling completely well these days, if you think about it for more than a second before you rush off to that next thing on your to-do list. It's nothing to put your finger on, just you're not feeling up to speed.

You look in the mirror and those love handles persist, your stomach won't shrink or tighten, and then there's the bloating, constipation, long sleepless nights, and this new overriding funk that comes and goes, but when it's there, it hangs over your head like a dark cloud. Where did that come from? You look in the mirror and you don't like what you see. You remember when your waist was tiny, even though you never realized (or appreciated) back then that you were small through the abdomen. You think, well, I'll just do more crunches; yes, that will do it. But it doesn't. Nothing seems to be working the way you'd like it to.

What happened? You used to be able to lose five pounds in a week if you really wanted to get into a favorite dress. Or you men go to button your pants and when you finally do, your gut flops over your pants and you have trouble tucking in your shirt. You used to be able to go to bed and know that you would sleep a good eight hours. What happened? When did you start sleeping five hours or less each night and restless sleep at that? And I'm sure you've heard that a lack of sleep makes you fat— which makes it all the harder not to stress about sleep!

Why is depression a new visitor to your life? Those blues go away with fattening foods, though, don't they?! Who cares? you ask yourself; what the heck, I'm fat, anyway, so let's pile on more bread, bagels, pasta, cakes, and cookies. That first bite makes you feel amazing, but then comes the self-loathing and more depression. Your friends who had really bad PMS used to have those terrible mood swings, but now you do, too. What happened?

And if you're like many, you may have noticed that you now react strangely to certain foods (like ice cream, which is now a guilty pleasure of the past unless you want your stomach to blow up like you are nine months pregnant). Come to think of it, pasta may not be sitting very well with you these days, either.

So what is different since you hit, or blew past, the halfway mark that is forty?

Before I explain, just know for starters that it's all fixable for you and your whole family. That's the good news. But to make the fixes stick, you have to commit to making some life changes or you will fail again and again.

To successfully lose fat after forty you need to understand the changes that have taken place on the planet that have created a toxic environment, and why and how these changes are affecting all of us. To unravel the solution to permanent weight loss that is unique to your age, you must understand that imbalanced hormones and chemicals play a huge part in the equation. *Huge!* Your age is a factor. You have been around long enough for the toxic buildup to have become a burden that you are constantly carrying in your body. This buildup creates a toxic load, and everything in your life is now affected by it.

With each of my books our collective knowledge grows, new elements about health reveal themselves, science makes more breakthroughs, and I get excited about sharing it all with you. *Sexy Forever* collects all that is current to give you updated information on permanent weight loss. I still follow all the tenets of weight loss that I have prescribed in past books, but now we are moving several steps farther in our ongoing education of how to stay thin, healthy, and happy. My new plan recognizes the changes in the planet that are affecting everyone.

Sexy Forever addresses why it is that you can't, or aren't, losing weight even though you are dieting. What exactly is wrong? Why is what you're doing no longer working for you?

We must accept that the world has changed. Toxicity is slowly killing us and these new changes in the environment, as well as our food supply and everyday stress, which is at an all-time high, are the reasons we've hit a wall not only in our wellness, but also in trying to lose weight. Now is the time to readjust how we handle these changes. The toxicity is not going away. But this book will show you how to live with it and not let it capsize your health and your weight.

Your grandparents had less stress, ate cleaner food, and their chemical exposure was nearly unheard of. Yet, as more and more of us were introduced to chemicals, we got sicker and fatter. Less than a hundred years ago "the big three"—cancer, heart disease, and diabetes—were relatively rare. Extreme obesity was reserved for the occasional circus performer. Why?

Something has to change. Sixty million people in America are obese! More than 9 million of them are ages six to nineteen years old. Our being overweight isn't solely attributable to the amount of food we are consuming. In fact, friends of mine who have serious weight problems appear to eat less than anyone else. They certainly eat less than I do. I have a very hearty appetite and I am able to maintain near perfect weight for my body composition.

> It's not just how much you are eating that is causing
> you problems, it is also *what* you are eating
> that is important.

Look at our children's diet. Our kids eat pizza for breakfast in elementary school! Worse yet, for lunch it's macaroni and cheese, a white-flour roll, and apple juice. Let's examine the foods offered to these children:

Pizza: trans fats, chemicals, white flour, and sugar (no nutrition)
Pepperoni: nitrates and chemicals (toxic)
Macaroni: white flour (no nutrition)

Cheese: from a macaroni package, man-made chemicals (toxic)

Apple juice: no fiber plus pesticides and added sugar (toxic)

This is not food! This is a nutrient-zero meal loaded with chemicals! How can we expect meals like these to build strong bodies and brains in our children? And the double jeopardy is setting them up for a lifetime of poor dietary choices. So much for a healthy diet! This is a disastrous diet, and these poor eating habits continue into adulthood, because these are the foods you grew up eating and they now have become your comfort foods.

Tragically, this is normal eating for Americans. As a people, we are fatter than any other country, and as my friend Dr. Burton Goldberg says:

"We are starving to death in the land of plenty!"

You aren't getting nutrition because of your toxic burden, and toxins are everywhere: in our food, water, household cleaners, and skin and hair care products. Ever wonder why you have chronic headaches, asthma, allergies, brain fog, fatigue, memory problems, depression, chronic pain, infections, and gut problems? I'm going to say this over and over in these pages. We are unknowingly filling our bodies with toxins that have burdened us, and sometimes these conditions are the body's way of screaming for help. It's not normal to have headaches or pain, or allergies or sinus or gut problems. These are signals to do something—and fast—because we are slowly killing ourselves. It's that important and that drastic. I am not shaking my finger at anyone here. It's not your fault. This situation has evolved, but the consequences are severe. And this book provides a clear alternative. *Stay with me.* Don't get overwhelmed. The solutions are coming.

The Iroquois Indians made decisions based on what impact they would have seven generations later. Ask yourself these questions: What do you think our country's present habits of eating poor-quality chemical-laden food will mean to our families in seven generations? Do you foresee perfect health? Do you see trim, toned bodies? Or do you see a lot of cancer, wheelchairs, obesity, mental disorders, Alzheimer's, heart disease, heart attacks, and chronic unrelenting diabetes? Perhaps you also see a loss of creativity and a dampening of the human spirit.

Some doctors are saying that the next generation will be sterile. Now whether or not you believe this will come to pass, you can at least see the possibilities from the effects of toxicity. It's no joke. It's serious and your weight is a language; a wake-up call from your body saying, "Do something *now!*"

It feels overwhelming: eliminate all the chemicals, eat real food. You wonder what is left for you to eat. How are you going to do this? Some people get very depressed when they learn of the toxic soup in which we live. *Stay with me.* Don't let it bring you down! Use this knowledge to make the changes where you can. Every little bit helps. I am extreme in attempting to remove toxins from my life and I know I am still surrounded. Do your best, but don't become overwhelmed and put on blinders to this reality you are about to discover. It's never been more important to educate yourself in order to rectify these environmental and age-related issues. If you don't start making changes now, the deterioration will begin. The longer you wait, the more difficult the job . . . but it's never impossible.

I am going to take you step-by-step through this process and show you the way. I have access to incredible doctors and experts who have shared their knowledge with me and I will now share it with you. You create your own course—and you would not have picked up this book unless you see yourself successful, healthy, and thin. When did it all change?

Food used to be more nutritious than it is today. The environment was cleaner. People exercised more each day just living their everyday lives. They didn't sit at their computers all day long. When it came to food, organic wasn't even a term. All food was organic. It wasn't until around the late 1950s when we began to liberally use poison sprays on our food that it became necessary to label food organic. Think how differently we'd react if they called food what it really has become: poisoned or not poisoned!

Which would you choose? Think about the craziness of the concept . . .
who decided it was a good idea to put poison on our food or spray chemicals around our homes?

Our food supply used to be loaded with essential nutrients that are being
depleted by modern-day agricultural methods. Nutrients that used to be in
our natural food supply now need to be taken as supplements. Previously,
we ate grass-fed beef with naturally occurring omega-3 fats. Today's corn-
fed beef, on the other hand, is loaded with hormones, antibiotics, and of
course excess omega-6 fats from the corn feed.

COMING CLEAN

In *Sexy Forever* you will learn that detoxing (cleaning out the body of
chemicals and toxins) will speed-dial in weight loss. The pounds are going
to fall off while you sit back and enjoy eating healthy, delicious food. Losing weight is truly not so much about portion control (although once
you've "cleaned house" and your body is receiving its nutritional requirements, you really won't crave as much food anymore). You will be fully
satisfied with the right amounts of food when the food you are taking in
is nutritious. A toxic body is not only extremely unhealthy, but also has a
slowed metabolism. A toxic body will cause you to get fatter and fatter,
while a cleansed one stays slim and, best of all, healthy.

GO WITH YOUR GUT

In this book I will be interviewing Brenda Watson, who is one of the foremost authorities on digestive health. Her specialties are healing the digestive system and saying goodbye to bloating and stomach discomfort.
Understanding gut health is crucial to your well-being. Gastrointestinal
(GI) disturbances are a primary cause of weight gain, and healing the gut
removes yet another obstacle to your goal. You will learn the importance
of probiotics and fiber as key secret weapons in weight loss. Fiber increases

the feeling of fullness, dampens hunger, and reduces caloric intake. You will also say goodbye to constipation, which plagues many adults and is an impediment to losing weight. Plus, you will learn about undetected food allergies or intolerances that may be keeping you bloated, puffy, overweight, or even chronically ill . . . and how a simple blood test can unravel these secrets and provide the easiest solution you could ever imagine to looking and feeling great.

THE BALANCING ACT

You can't lose weight if your hormones
aren't balanced.

Another key component to regaining your optimal weight and quality of life is to rebalance your hormones with natural bioidentical hormone replacement. You will hear from Dr. Jonathan Wright, the father of bioidentical hormones, and from Bill Faloon of Life Extension. They teach us that the balance of these important and vital hormones plays a significant role in determining not only our health, but also our weight. Why is it that when you were young and making a full complement of hormones you didn't battle weight as you do now?

It's your hormones!

Declining hormones create a cascade of bodily problems. Add to that the fact that stress further blunts hormone production and you get the picture.

The chemical exposure I have mentioned also blunts hormone production. And these factors lead to weight gain, accelerated aging, and poor health. Excess chemicals may also be the reason that hormones are declining at younger and younger ages with imbalances starting in our late thirties and early forties becoming much more common. This has never happened before.

Imbalanced hormones are a perfect setup not only for weight gain, but also disease. It is unfortunate that our medical schools do such a poor job educating our future physicians in hormone replacement. So often what are simply signs of hormonal decline are treated as a new "condition" for which a pharmaceutical appears to be the only answer. This is how more and more drugs creep into our lives. It's the middle-age dilemma affecting women *and* men. I have been replacing my declining hormones for fifteen years and every day is a good one. I am healthy, balanced, happy, and thin. My husband does it, too. It's not difficult, and I will explain how to do it. Once you connect the dots and absorb all of this new information, losing weight will become a breeze and, best of all, permanent.

> Losing weight permanently
> requires a commitment to change.

Being Sexy Forever requires new knowledge, a shift in your thinking, plus a commitment to making some permanent changes in your lifestyle and dietary habits. You have to approach this next passage in life differently.

Let's sum up what's true about fighting fat after forty:

- The reason you are having difficulty is environmental toxicity, which creates a toxic burden on your body and a change in your personal chemical makeup.

- Toxicity causes nutritional deprivation. Your body craves more and more food, trying to get what it needs to thrive.

- Hormonal disturbances cause accelerated aging, poor health, physical deterioration, and weight gain.

This lethal triad makes traditional dieting useless. It's no longer about eating less, it's about being smart about all the things that go in—and on—your body. In fact, once you discover the solution offered by *Sexy Forever* and hear what doctors and professionals have to say, you will understand how to decrease your toxic burden, you will master your cravings, and you will learn to fuel your body in a way that eliminates addictive eating. Once you understand the devastating effects of chemicals on your health, you will minimize where you can, live green, and choose foods that satisfy. You won't be left feeling hungry, and you will be thin and energetic.

Balancing your hormones will put you in a good mood, you will feel sexual once more, your brain will be sharp, your bones will be strong, and you can expect a blissful, deep sleep each night. I know this because after I made the simple changes I recommend in this book I was able to resolve a weight stall that had puzzled me. You, too, can discover which foods are causing problems and are an obstacle to weight loss and which foods will help instead of hurt. You will learn the benefits of herbs and spices that have antioxidant effects and help in eliminating the buildup of toxins that are causing the food cravings. Your meals will be absolutely scrumptious, and once you adapt to these changes you will be amazed that while you are on your way to being thin, sexy, and fabulous you will also be eating the greatest-tasting food of your life.

With the concepts of *Sexy Forever* you are going to make your insides young; and your healthy organs and glands will be operating at optimal levels. The effects created by these changes will make you youthful, healthy, and energetic naturally without any drugs.

The assault on our bodies from stress, aging, and toxicity is rectifiable. Hormonal imbalance raises insulin (the fat-storing hormone) levels and you get fatter. Toxins accumulate in the fat, requiring more and more fat to store them, depending on your particular personal makeup. Put the two elements together and you realize why, when you are eating only salads, you are getting fatter and fatter.

No more. You are about to begin a journey that will change your life.

Sexy Forever is *not* a diet. It's a new program for lifelong health and slimness. Diets don't work. Food is not the enemy. *Sexy Forever* offers a plan that clearly explains what you need to do and all you need to know.

PART I: WHAT'S MAKING— AND KEEPING—US FAT?

This section explains toxic buildup. Chemicals here, there, and everywhere are slowly causing more and more damage to you and it's insidious. It happens slowly, often without any of us really noticing. Little by little, it eats away at our once perfect health. It gets stored in the fat and is ready and waiting to attack when free-radical damage overwhelms your healthy cells and the immune system is compromised from an outside assault. Now you're in trouble.

When you ask yourself, Why are we so sick and why are we all so fat? I can only answer with another question: Why *wouldn't* we be sick and fat? Look at what we are doing to ourselves. What are we thinking? It took me some time to connect the dots, to really understand the devastating effects of toxins in our environment and poisons on our food. *Stay with me.* I will show you solutions to these problems so you can live a clean, healthy, long life with a slim body.

PART II: GOODBYE FAT, HELLO SEXY

This section provides an all-access pass to revered doctors, experts, and nutritionists who uncover obstacles that could be in your way.

You'll learn

- How to lessen toxic levels in your food and home; the importance of organic food, household cleaners, and skin care products (plus, how to manage if you can't afford organic).

- Balancing your hormones for health, wellness, sleep, sexuality, and weight loss.

- Digestive health—how you must heal your gut and uncover hidden allergies to have success losing weight.

- Exercise—you know me, I like it fast and easy. You can do this!

- Supplements—expert recommendations on what to take for health and weight loss.

PART III: THE EATING PLAN AND RECIPES

In this section we put the Sexy Forever weight loss plan into action. When it comes to food, the array you'll have available is vast and delicious. Real food is exciting. I don't eat boring food. My cooking is founded in Tuscan and country French, so I love a good wine reduction sauce or slow-cooked protein. The food choices and recipes I give you will be the best of your life. You can win this battle. It requires commitment, but it does not mean you are going to have to eat boring, portion-controlled meals. Ask any of my friends and they will tell you my food is fabulous (she says modestly). A few simple changes starting today will allow you to achieve your ideal body composition and stay that way. . . . deliciously.

You'll find

- The Detox Phase—the first thirty days designed to release the toxic burden and blast off those first pounds.

- Level 1 Weight Loss Phase—where you'll adopt a plan to enjoy incredible meals while you chisel down to your goal weight with your supercharged metabolism.

- Level 2 Lifestyle Phase—the maintenance plan where you learn to stay Sexy Forever!

- Jump-Start Your Success—outlining the most cutting-edge natural tools and products to make every step of the plan faster, easier, and more convenient. (I promise not to use the word *miracle*.)

- Recipes—delicious, all-new recipes, with menus for fabulous eating every day.

It's all here for you and yours for the taking. *Sexy Forever* is the answer to staying thin and healthy forever. Food is about to become your friend: delicious, fabulous, nutritious, incredible food! Get ready. Your life is about to transform. I will be with you every step of the way with additional support and resources at my online companion to this book SexyForeverPlan.com/book. *Stay with me* and imagine you . . . *Sexy Forever!*

PART I

What's Making—and Keeping—Us Fat?

THE TOXIC CONNECTION:
THE HEART OF THE PROBLEM

*For the first time in the history of the world, every human
being is now subjected to contact with dangerous chemicals,
from the moment of conception until death.*
                                    —RACHEL CARSON, *SILENT SPRING*

EXPERTS WEIGH IN:
WHAT ARE YOU UNKNOWINGLY TAKING IN?

Most of us are aware of toxins to which we are exposed in our food, water, and air; however, we are also surrounded by hidden ones. I asked Brenda Watson, author of *The Detox Strategy,* where else we are unknowingly taking them in. Her answer will shock you:

Let's begin with your bed. There are several ingredients that your body absorbs while you sleep, including toluene, a chemical linked to birth defects and emitted from the polyurethane foam that makes your bed so comfy, and perfluorooctanoic acid, a chemical that makes fabrics stain resistant but which is a hormone disruptor linked to ADHD in children. Then there are fire-retardant chemicals, some linked to learning disabilities and thyroid dysfunction, and some, like antimony, linked to heart and lung problems. As of July 1, 2007, all mattresses manufactured or imported into the United States must be treated with these fire-retardant chemicals. How about your carpet? Most likely it is synthetic and full of these same stain- and fire-resistant chemicals. When you brush your teeth, you know that warning label that says to keep your toothpaste out of reach of children under the age of six? Well, this label exists because your toothpaste exposes you to sodium fluoride, which is linked to enzyme disruption and thyroid problems. Also in your toothpaste may be sodium lauryl sulfate, which is linked to organ and reproductive toxicity, and triclosan, an antibacterial agent that's registered as a pesticide with the EPA and is linked to organ toxicity and possibly cancer. Most mouthwash contains formaldehyde and ammonia, several flavoring and coloring chemicals, as well as some chemicals that have leached from the plastic in the bottle. It's a huge problem, and difficult to minimize.

Depending on the type of shampoo and soaps you are using, you expose yourself to coloring agents, dyes, artificial preservatives, and propylene glycol, a suspected carcinogen. Most antiperspirants contain aluminum zirconium, which is toxic to the nervous and reproductive systems; a chemical called BHT, believed to be a hormone disruptor and neurotoxin; other chemicals that give the products their distinctive smell; and then there is more of that propylene glycol, linked to irritation and immune system toxicity.

If you dry-clean your clothes, you're exposed to a plethora of chemicals, including perchloroethylene (PCE), a chemical believed to be capable of causing cancer, especially in the liver and kidneys. It is also shown to affect developing fetuses. Even if you don't get your clothes dry-cleaned, what about synthetic fibers in your clothing (think polyester), which may be giving off small molecules of plasticizer fumes?

It goes on and on. It's in your makeup, cosmetics, hair spray (its ingredients can affect your nervous, reproductive, and immune systems), hair gel, mousse, and cream conditioner, which are equally toxic.

How did it get like this? How did our beautiful planet become so con-taminated? Our waters no longer run clean, our precious air is polluted, and oil has gushed into the Gulf of Mexico, contaminating our shores and our seafood. Chemicals are everywhere—in our homes, in our offices, in our gardens, and most unfortunately, in our bodies. And this toxicity is making us very unhealthy and very fat.

Remember this: you must be healthy to lose weight!

First, let's examine what the word *toxin* means. A toxin is a poisonous substance; it's taken from the Greek word *toxikon,* which means "arrow poison."

For our purposes, there are two types of toxins: environmental and internal. *Environmental* toxins include household chemicals, industrial pollutants, food additives, and pesticides. *Internal* toxins consist of waste products created by normal metabolic processes within the body. These toxins are produced as a result of our digestive system breaking down proteins, carbohydrates, and fats.

We are bombarded with external toxins: car exhaust, paint fumes, in-dustrial solvents, plasticizers, household cleaning products. Every breath we take is laden with tiny amounts of pollutants and poisons. I was hug-ging my little granddaughter the other day and I said, "You always smell so clean and fresh," but then I realized her clean clothes smelled like the laundry detergent and fabric softener her mom used, the same ones I had been using for so many years.

I used to spray my house with aerosol room fresheners and clean with foaming chemical cleansers; I used hair spray and tanning lotions and cos-metics laden with chemicals. We have all grown accustomed to the daily conveniences of modern life, but we don't make the connection between these and our unexplained weight gain and ailments. How about that new-car smell? You got it—it's a chemical. And it's making you fat.

Kids are now born with this crazy toxic burden, which is a tragedy. The researchers at the Environmental Working Group (EWG) examined the cord blood, which circulates between a baby and its mother's placenta, of infants born in U.S. hospitals to study how many toxins are passed on. The results were startling: the EWG found that newborns begin their lives with exposure to as many as 287 of the 413 toxic chemicals being studied. A range of between 154 and 231 toxins were found per baby, and 101 toxins were found in all of the babies. The 287 toxins included 180 chemical compounds that have been shown to cause cancer in either animals or humans.

Once we're born, we go on to accumulate tiny traces of poison every day. We have pollutants in the air we breathe both indoors and out, our food, our water, our soil, our backyards and gardens. Ever wonder how come you never see a bug in a grocery store? Ever wonder why you don't see insects or rodents in hotels, even with all the room service trays left around? Hmmmm . . . must be the chemical spray. Yes, supermarkets, hotels, and most places of business are routinely sprayed with pesticides, so that we never have to endure the sight of those little critters. But at what cost to our health?

We spray weedkillers like Round-Up as if they were some miracle. According to Dr. Russell Blaylock, renowned neuroscientist and one of my dear friends, "The 'miracle' is that there is an 800 percent increased risk of multiple myeloma [a cancer of the white blood cells] connected with users of Round-Up." In Los Angeles, Department of Recreation and Parks trucks proudly state on the sides, "We use Round-Up!" They are spraying it everywhere, and we are breathing it, walking through it, sitting on green lawns covered in it, playing in it, and worst of all, contaminating our food with it.

According to Brenda Watson in her book *The Detox Strategy,* "Our diets and health are unfortunately largely controlled by three giant sectors and driving forces of the economy: food and agricultural corporations, including processed food giants; pharmaceutical companies; and the chemical and manufacturing industry, which aims to create unnaturally occurring products that may be superior in some ways to naturally occurring ones, yet incredibly harmful to humans in other ways. Because these three sectors are huge economic generators we are led to believe their activities are okay, that processed and chemically altered or modified foods and agriculture, as well as chemically engineered goods and drugs, are actually better than what nature would provide. But this is far from the truth. They may be better in the sense that they make our lives easier, but the cost is exposure to potentially harmful substances."

There are many of us saying the same thing. We are noticing what has happened. We are noticing that business is in control of our environment, our food, and our health. But the majority of the population is in a fog. In this case, ignorance is not bliss. And wearing blinders to the dangers of toxicity is to invite disease, obesity, and a shortened life.

Let's talk about some of the areas where ignorance is leading us to dangerous grounds. Take fluoride. How did its widespread use come about? Fluoride is a huge problem for humans despite what the American Dental Association (ADA) has to say about it. It's crucial to install reverse osmosis filters on all your faucets, including in showers and bathtubs, for protection, but fluoride eats away at the filters, so they must be changed every three months. If fluoride does that to a filter in three months, imagine what it is doing inside your body! "You have to understand it's all a payoff system," says Dr. Russell Blaylock. "Fluoride is a waste product. Communities keep trying to refuse it, and they come back every year and try again. They offer cities contracts, government contracts, and dangle the possibility that they are going to do a big project if this community agrees to fluoridate the water supply.

"Fluoride is one of the most poisonous substances on earth. It tends to accumulate in the body, particularly in the bones, thyroid gland, and brain. It lowers IQ. It's associated with Down syndrome, and it triggers toxicity in the human body. But the people who are promoting it (primarily the government and the ADA) have so much influence through the media that you really can't get the truth out. People are just not aware how enormously toxic fluoride is, particularly when combined with aluminum. When you mix them together, which is what happens in drinking water, they combine chemically and form a substance that acts as a false transmitter for what are called G protein receptors in brain cells, as well as other cells, and wreak all kinds of havoc. We also find that some tumor cells have these G-type receptors, some of which are glutamate (chemical) receptors, and that fluoride activates them." So this connects to the findings that fluoride increases cancer growth and cancer mortality. Plus, its toxicity to your body makes you fat. Imagine—you can get fat from your drinking water.

PCBs (polychlorinated biphenyls) are another major source of our toxic burden and need to be eliminated from our bodies. PCBs are highly toxic chemicals found in adults and also in the cord blood of newborns! PCBs were originally manufactured for use as coolants in electrical transformers, and then they went on to serve many other industrial uses. Because they were found to be so toxic and dangerous to our health, PCBs have been banned worldwide since the 1970s. Yet they are so persistent in the environment that they are still found in fish, animals, and people. For example, they are found in cattle feed, which then makes its way into the cow, then into the milk and meat, and ultimately into human stomachs.

Stay with me. Solutions are on the way, but having knowledge is vital!

> In global samplings of butter, the highest levels of
> PCBs have been found in butter made in Europe and
> North America.

WHAT ABOUT PLASTICS?

For the sake of convenience we have enjoyed the ease and convenience of nonstick pots and pans, and we have untold ways of using plastic in the kitchen, from soft sandwich bags to hard storage containers and bottles.

These conveniences make modern life much easier than it once was, but again, at what cost to our health?

Bisphenol A (BPA) is an ingredient used to make a wide variety of plastic goods and to line metal food and drink cans (that's why those canned products slip so easily out of the can). The convenience is hardly worth this toxin, which is associated with birth defects of the male and female reproductive systems. What is troubling is that BPA is unregulated, allowed in unlimited amounts in consumer products, drinking water, and food.

Our Teflon-coated pots and pans have been touted as the nonstick miracle, but unfortunately the toxins from Teflon stay forever in the environment and in your body. When Teflon is heated, the chemicals emitted into the air will kill some birds if they are in the same room. What do you suppose this off-gassing is doing to us?

Aluminum also has been linked to Alzheimer's, as it is a powerful neurotoxin that damages brain cells. Yet it is found in a number of our everyday products, including the vaccines given regularly to children. Almost all water and food contain some form of aluminum, as it is used by municipal water supplies as a flocculating agent to remove dirt. It is also widely used in food processing, foil and utensils, antiperspirants, paints, cosmetics, and baking powders as well as over-the-counter painkillers, anti-inflammatory drugs, antacids, and douche preparations (ouch!).

Look in your kitchen right now and see how many of these products you use on a daily basis. You will start to see the enormous size of the toxic burden we are all carrying in our bodies, residing in our fat. Think of your most-stuffed storage closet. What do you do when you can't fit any more in it? You enlarge the closet to hold all the contents. That's what is happening to you. The more toxins you take in, the more fat is required to store them.

TOXIC OVERLOAD

> *A little knowledge (which is what we call ignorance) is, in*
> *fact, a dangerous thing. Almost everyone, at least in the*
> *industrialized world, knows that drinking water from a filthy*
> *pond or polluted lake can cause life-threatening diarrhea, but*
> *still only a few realize that holding on to resentment, anger,*
> *and fear, or eating fast foods, chemical additives, and artificial*
> *sweeteners, is no less dangerous than drinking polluted water;*
> *it may just take a little longer to kill a person than a tiny*
> *amoeba can.*
>
> —ANDREAS MORITZ

Major ailments are now so commonplace that we pay little attention to how widespread they have become: asthma, diabetes, fibromyalgia, infertility, Parkinson's disease, bone cancer, leukemia, and lymphoma, as well as autoimmune diseases such as lupus, rheumatoid arthritis, and Hashimoto's thyroiditis.

Toxin-induced sicknesses are growing like weeds. Yet we haven't connected the dots. Toxins make us fat and make us sick, and are the missing piece to the puzzle of why we can't lose weight and why we feel so lousy. Where is the tipping point? What chemical, what fume, what pesticide, what toxin is the one that puts you over the top?

Obesity rates have more than doubled in the past thirty years. Doesn't it raise the question of why? Toxins make you fat. It's that simple, and that complex. Here's why.

Mitochondria are the little powerhouses inside every living cell in your body. They provide power for your cells by creating energy from fats and sugars, thereby driving your metabolism and fueling your whole body.

When toxins enter your body the buildup damages the mitochondria, your cellular power plants, so they no longer work effectively. As a result, fats and sugars that aren't being burned for fuel pile up all over the body in the form of extra pounds. Also, without the mitochondria working optimally, you lose your physical energy. You see it every day—middle-aged people who are out of gas, have no energy, always feel sluggish. Is that you? If so, you probably don't have the energy to exercise, and this fatigue causes food cravings, usually for sugar and carbohydrates. So now there's a domino effect—but you are the one getting knocked down, while you get fatter and fatter.

> Every one of us is living in a toxic world.

We are under the greatest environmental assault in the history of mankind. Toxins are everywhere; they're in our homes, our offices, the air we breathe, the water we drink, the food we consume, the cosmetics and creams we put on our bodies. Just by living in this day and age we build up a toxic load. These toxins move throughout the bloodstream alongside the nutrients, the oxygen and other essentials, our bodies need. These man-made chemicals, originally designed to help us live better lives, were never intended to be inside of us. At some point these toxins reach critical mass in our bodies, and then we're in trouble. What microwaved food covered in plastic, or diet soda, or trans-fat-laden fast-food burger, or pesticide will be the tipping point to toxic overload and an entrée to disease and obesity?

BEAST OF BURDEN

Americans' average toxic burden is higher than it's ever been. And the obesity rate in this country is off the charts. So connect the dots. It's not a coincidence. Scientific studies show a strong correlation between levels of toxic burden, higher body weight, and the risk of diabetes.

Yet not all people who carry a toxic burden are fat. Some people are better at fighting back, but this toxic load will surface in ways other than obesity: fatigue, autoimmune diseases such as lupus or fibromyalgia, cancer, allergies, and food intolerances to wheat, gluten, dairy, and sugar.

Toxic overload comes on slowly, one day at a time, one year at a time, with the symptoms creeping up and getting worse and worse. It starts with relatively benign things like exhaustion, and then more serious conditions erupt such as asthma, gut disturbances, food intolerances, depression, arthritis, heart disease, cancer, Parkinson's, and diabetes. These are all terrible conditions and diseases that are debilitating to the human body.

NOWHERE TO RUN

No matter how the toxins get into our bodies, whether through the lungs, stomach, or skin, they all meet the liver at some point and from there get sent to the kidneys and colon for elimination, become trapped in bones, muscles, tissues, or other organs, or they get locked in the liver itself, *or* they get stored away in fat cells!

The fact that many toxins get trapped in fat cells deserves special attention. Fat cells don't get broken down easily, so the toxins literally weigh the body down. If you carry excess fat, burning up that fat releases toxins into the bloodstream for proper removal. As toxins accumulate, they act in unsuspected ways. You begin to experience health problems like allergies, colds, migraines, and infertility, or major diseases like breast cancer and dementia.

Avoiding fat-soluble toxins sounds like a solution, but it is very difficult to do. We are constantly exposed to fat-soluble toxic chemicals used as solvents, glues, paints, or cleaning products. Toluene and benzene are solvents (meaning they are capable of dissolving other substances) that we typically encounter in daily life when we pump gas, shop for clothes, buy a new car, or pick up the dry cleaning.

These fat-soluble chemicals collect in the fatty tissues of the body rather than being excreted quickly. They are particularly damaging to people who are deficient in nutrients called essential fatty acids, because a body deprived of essential fats is a body that will grab on to most any oily substances, even toxic substances like diesel fuel! These compounds can cause liver and kidney damage as well as skin irritation. This information is depressing, right? I know I sound like doom and gloom in contrast to my usual optimistic self. Stay with me. Solutions are coming, but first, know thy enemy.

It is clear that daily exposure to toxins makes us ill. Some people will develop conditions sooner than others, but if you do not change your diet and lifestyle, toxicity will most likely affect you at some point. But there is another dimension to the definition of what is a toxin that is frequently overlooked. And substances you wouldn't normally view as toxic or poisonous absolutely can be: pharmaceutical drugs, excessive caffeine, even alcohol. I point this out so you don't deceive yourself that things like over-the-counter painkillers and tequila are good for you. They are instead toxic to our system; they are foreign substances to the body, especially your liver, which has to process all of them. A cup of coffee a day and the occasional glass of red wine or tequila shooter can be handled by the body *if* the toxic burden you are carrying is under control. We are going to learn how to reduce this burden on your body so that these pleasures can be enjoyed.

DETOX FOR HEALTH

Detoxification is a constant bodily process. We are continually eliminating toxins through our digestive, urinary, skin, circulatory, respiratory, and lymphatic systems. Nature is wondrous and has thought it all out for us. These systems are brilliant, but sad to say, these marvelous systems are being taxed to the point of near uselessness by the chemical onslaught of today's world. We regularly consume poor-quality food contaminated by pesticides and animal proteins that have been injected with chemicals such as antibiotics and growth hormones. As a result, people today are sick and fat, with detoxification systems that just are not able to cope.

The word *detoxification* also relates to the treatments employed to help support the function of these natural detoxification channels. In this sense detoxification is about taking an active role in stimulating your body's innate ability to cleanse itself.

Most people think of colon cleansing as the only way to detoxify, but this is a very narrow view. Detoxing is not about taking a laxative and going on with your poor diet and lifestyle habits. It's about doing internal cleanses on a regular basis, changing your diet to healthy, nonpoisonous (organic) food, using fresh herbs and spices as natural antioxidants, and switching out household cleaners to green nontoxic ones. The more you reduce your toxic burden, the faster you will experience improved health and a thinner body. Toxins are very difficult to eliminate, and you have to make a concerted effort to reduce your personal toxic burden if you are to have true hope for success.

WHY A HEALTHY LIVER IS KEY TO LOSING WEIGHT

Body fat accumulation, especially around the midsection, suggests that your liver is not functioning as efficiently as it could. Detoxification is the way to a healthy liver—and a slim waistline.

When your liver works efficiently, it's much easier to lose weight. If your liver gets overloaded, increased levels of toxins will be circulating in your blood, and those toxins can damage your organs and glands and interfere with their ability to function properly. Toxicity confuses your body and creates poor health. As a result, you cannot metabolize well, you will have no energy, you will not absorb nutrients essential to life, and you won't be able to fight disease. If your liver is sluggish and bile production is insufficient, instead of breaking down fat and processing it your liver stores it away, usually in a big spare tire around your middle. Constant stress on the liver interferes with both bile production and detoxification, leading to stress, fatigue, weight gain, and toxic buildup inside your body.

So what puts extra stress on your liver and interferes with your liver's ability to efficiently detoxify? Here is a list of just a few of the most common culprits:

- Sugar and artificial sweeteners.

- Trans-fatty acids (found in partially hydrogenated oils). Partial hydrogenation of vegetable oil is a process that turns healthy oils into essentially "plastic" oil and creates killer trans-fatty acids.

- Most over-the-counter pain relievers and practically all prescription drugs, including blood pressure medications and cholesterol-lowering drugs.

- Regular alcohol consumption. Two servings (preferably of red wine) a couple of times a week is fine; more than that becomes toxic to your system. Look for organic wine as a best choice, sold at stores like Whole Foods.

- Constipation. If the colon is backed up, the liver dumps the toxins into the cells and the toxins build up in the body. Regular colonics, enemas, or coffee enemas are good ways of irrigating the colon and cleaning out constipation.

Therefore, if during any given day you put artificial sweetener in your coffee, eat at a fast-food restaurant, take an Advil, pop down your daily Lipitor prescription, and are constipated from toxins and lack of exercise, then accept that you have totally messed with the natural function of your liver, your vital detoxification organ. Most Americans are doing this on a daily basis. And we wonder why we are sick and fat!

When you couple your toxic burden with hormonal imbalance, the combination is a setup for weight gain and disease.

> If you are overweight, you are not healthy. If you are
> *not* hormonally balanced, you are not healthy.

If you consume, live with, breathe, or bathe in chemicals, you are not healthy, and that pretty much includes everyone on the planet. Not to worry. I have a plan for detoxing and losing weight.

WHAT *ARE* WE EATING?

Food is now nothing more than plastic for people's mouth entertainment.

—DR. STEVEN NELSON

Family meals are a ritual of the past. Now instead, children graze or forage; but unlike previous hunter gatherers, they do not come up against a scarcity of food, but rather a surfeit of it. Nothing is easier for them than to overindulge, and the appetite grows with the feeding. Their tastes never develop beyond the most instantly gratifying types of food; sugary and fatty, and they eat like children for the rest of their lives.

—*WALL STREET JOURNAL*

We now know that chemicals are everywhere and that they are insidious. The toxic load they put on the body is awful, but there is another reason they impede weight loss. Here it is: our bodies crave nutrients, yet we eat foods and so-called diet foods that have no real nutritional value. This leaves us craving more and more of this bad food, and as a result we eat more and more chemicals and more and more preservatives. We ignorantly consume genetically modified foods, not realizing that these foods are void of nutrition and can lead to weight gain and disease.

> No one knows the long-term dangers
> of these new engineered foods.

Why do we keep trying to outthink Mother Nature?

Look at corn and soy. They are some of the top genetically modified crops. You think you're choosing a healthy alternative, but you're not. All genetically modified (GM) soy contains fat, which is a great carrier of toxins. A high soy intake has been linked with lower thyroid function, so if you are switching to soy products for health and weight loss, it could actually be working against you.

Before we go further, it might help to know what I mean by genetically modified foods. These are foods that have been genetically altered to withstand spraying with pesticides or to introduce other new characteristics. In modifying the seed, we don't know what other effects might result. Might the modification produce new toxins? Trigger allergies? Increase antibiotic resistance? In a recent study of rats fed a diet exclusively of genetically modified foods, all the rats developed organ damage, and many died.

In the movie *Food Inc.*, writer Michael Pollan says, "The way we eat has changed more in the last fifty years than in the previous ten thousand. You go into the supermarket and you see pictures of farmers, the picket fence, the silo, the thirties farmhouse, and the green grass. It's the spinning of this pastoral fantasy. The American supermarket has on average forty-seven thousand products. There are no seasons in the American supermarket. Now there are tomatoes all year round, grown halfway around the world, sprayed with pesticides, picked when they were green, and ripened with ethylene gas." It's the same with strawberries, bananas . . . and the list goes on and on.

This is just the beginning. Until recently we just didn't think about things like pesticides and ethylene gas. How are these new chemicals affecting our health? We are now engineering our foods so that they don't go bad in the refrigerator or become rancid as quickly. But at what price to us?

Corn is the main ingredient in feed for chicken, hogs, and cattle. It's cheap. In the United States today, 30 percent of our agricultural land base is being planted with corn, largely driven by government policy. High-fructose corn syrup (HFCS) can be found in virtually everything, and since its introduction in the 1950s, it has been one of the main contributors to the incredible rise in diabetes here.

> More smoke and mirrors:
> The food industry is trying to change
> high-fructose corn syrup's name to "corn sugar."
> Be on the lookout; it's the same bad stuff.

According to Pollan, "Corn is the great raw material. You get that big fat kernel of starch and break it down and reassemble it." This is how they make high-fructose corn syrup; it is also where we get maltodextrin, diglycerides, and many of the other unpronounceable ingredients in processed food that we've become so used to seeing. They are now part of everyday life. We have to understand how widespread this is to grasp the profound effect chemicals are having on our health and the rise in obesity.

When you go to a supermarket, what looks like a cornucopia of choice is not. There is an illusion of diversity, but actually there are only a few large companies involved, and so much of our industrial food turns out to be clever rearrangements of corn.

Corn has conquered the world in a lot of ways. It is a remarkable plant, and land that used to produce 20 bushels of corn an acre can now produce 200 bushels an acre, which is an astonishing achievement for breeders (I wouldn't call them farmers any longer). Chemical fertilizers also deserve credit, as do pesticides.

But again I ask: at what cost to us is this remarkable achievement? Disease and obesity are at all-time highs. A diet of high-fructose corn syrup and refined carbohydrates leads to spikes of insulin and gradually a wearing down of the system by which our body metabolizes sugar.

We're now even feeding corn to fish. Whether we are eating farmed tilapia or salmon, we're eating corn. Think about it—we are teaching fish to eat corn, and cattle have been retrained to go against their natural evolutionary inclinations to eat grass. Now we are feeding them corn to fatten them up cheaply. Yes, corn is high in starch and is fattening—*very fattening*—and our protein is being fed a diet of it. Then we are eating that animal, which fattens *us* up. Add to that the numerous products we all have on our pantry shelves loaded with corn derivatives, and you get the picture.

The industrial food system is always looking for greater efficiency, but many new steps in efficiency lead to problems. One result: feed corn to cattle and the dangerous *E. coli* O157:h7 bacterium hits the world stage. How does this happen? It's their new diet of corn, which is not natural for cattle, giving them infections and making them less healthy (and since they are not getting the proper nutrients, we don't either). Combine that with the overuse of antibiotics and the filth in feedlots where cattle stand ankle deep in their manure all day long, and it's a recipe for disaster. When these feces-covered cattle are sent to the slaughterhouse, they are thrown on top of each other, and contaminated meat gets mixed up with noncontaminated meat. That's how *E. coli* gets into our meat supply. Remember the poor little boy who died from *E. coli*–tainted meat from a Jack in the Box? This is the meat that ends up in fast-food restaurants, the food of choice for the majority of Americans.

Gone are the pastures with cows lazily grazing on natural green grass. Recently I drove up Highway 101 from southern California to Big Sur for one of my favorite vacations, a stay at the Post Ranch Inn. Along the way I was pleased and delighted to see gently rolling hills covered with beautiful green grass, where brown and white cows were happily grazing. In describing this pastoral scene to a supplier I work with, I proudly pointed out that I had been touched by this beautiful scene. What she said shocked me: "I know it looks perfect, but regrettably, this is not the end stage; this is just a temporary stop on their way to the feedlots. Most all American cows are sent to the feedlots, and once they get there, they are all shoved together with no room to move. Then they are force-fed corn to fatten them up. There's more money in fat cows. It's pretty difficult to find grass-fed cows in the United States anymore."

> Did you know that many countries ban American beef? According to CNN, Singapore, Malaysia, Taiwan, Japan, and South Korea have all banned U.S. beef imports at some time in the last decade.

Yet according to Michael Pollan, if you take cattle off their corn diet, within five days they will shed 80 percent of the dangerous strain of *E. coli* in their gut. But does the cattle industry do this? No. Instead they use ammonium hydroxide to try to kill it. Ammonia kills bacteria, but it doesn't get to the root of the problem. The end result is more chemicals for us—plus the added bonus of more disease and more obesity.

Imagine.

We need nutrients for survival. To be healthy and thin, we need real food that has not been sprayed with poison or had its genes tinkered with. Unfortunately, genetically modified foods are not labeled as such in the United States. That is why organic food is the healthy choice—truly, the only real *food* choice.

Harmful foods have invaded our pantries without most of us ever realizing that by consuming them *we* are playing a huge part in contributing to the epidemic of obesity and poor health. Think about the craziness of this. The world is on a low-fat craze, yet obesity, heart disease, diabetes, and cancer are at an all-time high! Obviously what we have been doing isn't working. Low-fat foods, diet foods, and foods laden with chemicals are not the answer.

The body operates on nutrients. They are essential to life and health. You can't be healthy if you are not getting the proper nutrients, which includes healthy oils. But things have gone so wrong in today's world, and these changes are tragic for us.

Food is nowhere near as nutritious and nutrient-dense as it used to be. For instance, take apples. According to the U.S. Department of Agriculture, apples today have fewer minerals than apples grown in 1990. That means you have to eat more apples to get the same nutritional value your grandparents received from eating just one! This is only one example. Our fruits and vegetables are now largely grown in mineral-depleted soil, so the nutrient content is dramatically reduced compared to before. Because of this, our bodies now require proper supplementation to get the needed minerals and vitamins.

Essential nutrients play a big role in everything about your health, including your ability to burn stored body fat and maintain a healthy weight. If you don't get enough of the essential vitamins and minerals to enable your organs and glands to function properly, your health will suffer. Weight gain and degenerative disease are connected; a lack of nutrients combined with the slowdown of our metabolisms creates hormonal imbalance and sets our bodies up for disease. Unfortunately, not much attention is paid to mineral deficiency in orthodox medicine. Yet replacement helps to speed up the weight loss process, with the bonus of better health.

DRINKING IN OUR FAT

News flash: Artificial sweeteners make you fat!

There is no such thing as "junk food," only "junk diets"!
—DR. HELEN A. GUTHRIE

Ever wonder why people who walk around all day drinking diet sodas are not thin? The average diet soda addict drinks anywhere from a six-pack to a case of diet soda *daily*. Because diet sodas are made from chemicals, there are no nutrients for the body to extract, and this confuses the brain, whose job it is to look at all food as building blocks. When you drink diet soda, the brain finds nothing recognizable as nutrition to make healthy cells; as a result, the brain tries again and again to get fed, triggering cravings for more. When you are depleted because of toxicity, you tend to go for sugars and carbohydrates . . . or more diet sodas. This results in more and more chemicals and further activates cravings for foods that make you fat.

Diet sodas make you crave fattening foods.

I was appalled when the makers of soft drinks decided to oblige the First Lady's campaign to end childhood obesity by banning sugared soft drinks from vending machines in schools. Why? Surely it's great to get rid of the soda . . . except the sugared versions are being replaced by diet sodas! The chemicals in diet sodas have been directly linked to the worst kinds of brain tumors and are major contributors to obesity.

According to Dr. Russell Blaylock, "There is powerful evidence that MSG and other excitotoxic chemical food additives [such as the artificial sweetener aspartame] induce extreme obesity that lasts a lifetime (it's re-lated to a loss of leptin receptors in the hypothalamus). Recent studies have also shown that aspartame induces obesity in a number of people, probably for the same reason. The rise in childhood obesity is accompa-nied by a rise in metabolic syndrome, which is also produced by early life exposure to MSG and probably aspartame. Often forgotten is that soy contains high levels of glutamate and can trigger similar reactions as MSG. Because so many children have been exposed to high levels of MSG, as they age we see a large number of people from fifty on with uncontrollable obesity. The characteristic of this form of obesity is that it is very difficult to remove with dieting and is quite resistant to exercise. The astronomical rise in type 2 diabetes is in large part secondary to early MSG exposure, and when combined with the massive intake of HFCS [high-fructose corn syrup] and simple sugars, the rates go up even higher. Stopping the excitotoxin exposure is vital for ending obesity and for the sake of health for all people."

According to J. J. Virgin in *Six Weeks to Sleeveless and Sexy,* "In a recent study, rats were given sugar water and then rat food. They ate what they needed to maintain their weight. Then the same rats were given artifi-cially sweetened water, and again they ate what they needed to maintain their weight. The problem arose when the rats went back to drinking the sugar water, as they could no longer correlate the degree of sweetness with the amount of calories, so they overate." When you eat sweet, you crave sweet. As this author points out, "If you are trying to retrain your taste buds to perceive a blueberry or an apple as delicious and sweet, it will be impossible to do so if you keep confusing your taste buds to think that artificially supersweetened jam is the level of sweetness that sets the bar." Again, not to worry. I will provide several natural sweetening solu-tions in the coming chapters.

In order for a product to be labeled
"artificial sweetener," it must contain chemicals—
stay away from them!

MYTH: TOXINS ARE HARMLESS IN SMALL AMOUNTS

At this point in your life, your body is weighed down by a toxic burden and cannot handle any more chemicals. Fresh organic food is the best place to start healing, and in eating it you feed the little powerhouses (mitochondria) that fuel your weight loss and every vital system in your body. Say goodbye to the chemicals and poisons you have unconsciously taken in until now.

Unfortunately, we will never again be able to live an existence that is devoid of chemicals and toxins unless we move to the most remote part of the globe and eliminate all modern conveniences and technologies from our lives, and even then acid rain and chemical-laden clouds would likely be passing overhead. But don't be overwhelmed. Simple changes add up, creating an internal environment predominantly made up of healthy cells rather than unhealthy cells. This new ratio will change your health, and as a result the pounds will drop away. Having a high ratio of healthy cells to malfunctioning cells is a key to beating the present unavoidable environmental assault. And it's key to staying Sexy Forever.

We can get fat because of overeating and lack of exercise, but in middle age we now know there's more to it. When we're overweight we feel fatigued, but this fatigue and the accompanying fat are, as we have established, a result of environmental toxins. It's the toxins that make it *impossible* for your body to absorb nutrients. When you don't absorb nutrients, your body is essentially starving, which makes you hungry for more and more food. But the body can't get what it needs because of this devastating toxic burden. This cycle will not stop without intervention, and as a result, you will gain more and more weight.

Without nutrients the body begins to decline in many ways. If you reduce your load of toxins, you will have more energy and fewer pounds of fat. When you start absorbing nutrients again, you won't crave poor-quality foods, and you will start gravitating to foods that have high nutritional content. The body is smart, but it can't help you out when chemicals are blocking all entryways for nutrition. Imagine trying to run your car without gas.

But just getting rid of the fat doesn't get rid of the toxins. They are re-absorbed into your body and new fat *immediately* starts to collect. This is what creates the vicious cycle.

HELLO TV DINNERS, GOODBYE HEALTH

We need to retrain ourselves to eat as we were meant to eat. I believe one of the ways we got started on this path was with TV dinners. When I was a kid, I used to beg my mother to buy TV dinners. I thought they were a treat, but when you actually think about it, TV dinners are a form of poison. Let's just start with the aluminum trays, which we heated on high. (If you recall, you used to be able to taste the aluminum.) So right there you have a big dose of heavy metals, which have been linked to brain tumors, among many other things. The food itself was of poor quality and non-nutritious. The oils used were bad. And the most exciting part of the meal was the gooey, sugary, apple-y, chemical-y thing they called dessert.

TV dinners began our transition from real nutrition to toxic, chemical-filled food, and the obesity rate rose commensurately, as did rates of diabetes, heart disease, and cancer.

Don't be afraid of real food. If you want to stay Sexy Forever, first and most important, you must eat real food—in other words, foods that come from nature, not man-made foods, not fake foods, not any foods with chemicals.

BECOME AWARE OF FOOD ADDITIVES

You must also become informed about food additives. Harmful gluta-mates such as MSG may be hidden in food ingredients such as caseinate, autolyzed yeast enzymes, beef or chicken broth, natural flavorings, soy protein, hydrolyzed protein, soy isolates, and soy protein concentrates. This is how large manufacturers get around listing MSG. (That being said, these ingredients do not always contain MSG.) If you are truly serious about losing weight and getting healthy, you must be vigilant about avoiding these substances.

WHAT WE SHOULD BE EATING: BUTTER AND OTHER GOOD FATS

It is important to become knowledgeable about good and bad fats. The wrong choice of fats will have a serious effect on your health and your ability to lose weight.

> Omega-3 fats are heart-healthy fats.

The right choices of fats are crucial to the membranes of every one of the trillions of cells in your body. Omega-3 fats create a soft, pliable membrane around each cell, allowing for water and air (hydration and oxygenation) to flow through. *Life* is water and air, and the good omega-3 oils that promote life are perilla oil, flaxseed oil, and fish oil. Animal fats from healthy animals like grass-fed cattle are also acceptable in moderation; it is a shame these healthy, naturally occurring fats have been demonized by the food processing industry.

When your cells have the proper amounts of water and oxygen, the mitochondria (the energy source of your cells) work optimally, and a side benefit is rapid weight loss. Well-functioning hydrated cells also reverse the aging process and create a smoothly functioning, healthy body. When water and air are not penetrating the cells, your energy slows or stops, resulting in potentially serious effects on your health, all while setting you up to get fatter and fatter.

> Trans fats and too many omega-6 fats are harmful.

Trans fats found in partially hydrogenated oils, margarine, and shortening are the worst type of fats because they are completely unnatural. Less
known are the dangers of omega-6 fats, which are found in safflower oil,
sunflower oil, corn oil, peanut oil, soybean oil, cottonseed oil, among others. Too many omega-6 fats and not enough omega-3 fats creates a hard
membrane around each cell, like an eggshell. Free radicals entering your
body can cause the membrane to crack, and now you have a malfunctioning cell. When you reach a point where you have more malfunctioning
cells than healthy cells, you will most likely become very ill, possibly with
diseases such as cancer and heart disease. Along the way your weight will
soar. A simple step such as changing the oils you consume can positively
impact the health of your cells; there is no drug that can do that.

I think Sally Fallon in her book *Nourishing Traditions* says it best:
"During the sixty-year period from 1910 to 1970, the proportion of traditional animal fat in the American diet declined from 83 percent to
62 percent, and butter consumption plummeted from 18 pounds per
person per year to four. During the past eighty years, dietary cholesterol
intake has increased only 1 percent. During the same period the percentage of dietary vegetable oils in the form of margarine, shortening and refined oils increased about 400 percent while the consumption of sugar
and processed foods increased about 60 percent." Americans are dying of
heart disease from sugar, processed foods, bad oils, margarine, shortening, and refined foods. We are getting fatter and fatter eating all this poor-
quality food.

WHAT WE SHOULD BE EATING:
MORE PROTEIN

Overall, we need high-quality protein at most every meal. By high-quality, I mean protein that has not been contaminated by chemicals, pesticides, growth hormones, or antibiotics. Protein is extremely important and is involved in every life function from your bone marrow to your skin. Proteins are found in both animal and vegetable sources. Animal-source protein is complete protein because almost all animal proteins contain all eight essential amino acids in optimal proportions. This ratio of amino acids is very valuable to your body.

Studies prove that too little protein in your body results in health problems that range in severity from a suppressed immune system and physical weakness to stunted growth and mental retardation. It takes a diet of at least 30 percent protein to maximize the biochemicals (eicosanoids) in your system that enhance your immune system, decrease inflammation and pain, increase oxygen flow, improve endurance, and more.

Fish is a great source of protein. Chicken and beef are a great source of protein but chicken should be organic and beef grass-fed whenever possible; conventionally raised poultry may suffer from the same problems of poor-quality feed and overcrowding that conventionally raised cattle and pigs do. Russia doesn't want our chicken, and they have a food shortage. That should tell you something!

> Russia, along with several other countries, has banned poultry from the United States because of the chlorine (a known carcinogen) used in the processing.

Besides, organic chickens taste so much better. If you cannot afford organic, look for natural poultry and meats raised without antibiotics or hormones. These are always better choices and will contribute to your daily health and nutritional requirements.

DETOX FIRST, LOSE WEIGHT AFTER

Losing weight without getting rid of the toxins ensures that you *will* gain back all the fat and more. Think about it—just getting rid of the fat doesn't get rid of the toxins, which are reabsorbed into your body. This creates a vicious cycle. Losing weight without learning to eliminate chemicals is like a merry-go-round. And it's why dieting doesn't work. Plus the toxic load makes it more and more difficult for people from age forty on to lose weight.

Now do you understand why losing weight has been a frustrating battle for you? Are you ready to get off that not-so-merry-go-round?

Here we go!

PART II

Goodbye Fat, Hello Sexy

CLEAN UP YOUR ACT

*The need to tackle toxic burdens before they manifest
themselves as disease has never been greater. It is clear that
the future of health care will have at its very core an absolute
requirement for safe and effective detoxification procedures,
hopefully instituted before the individual's immune system and
vital organs have ceased to operate adequately.*

—DR. LEON CHAITOW

The goal of *Sexy Forever* is to enhance and improve your overall health, give your body what it craves, and help you remain toxin free and in peak condition for life. In doing this you will be rewarded with a thin, beautiful body. Recapturing health through detoxification is more than possible—it's within your reach. But what does detox mean?

Detoxing means avoiding chemicals as best you can:

- In your food

- In your household cleaning products

- In your cosmetics

- In shampoos and conditioners

- In your bath, shower, or pool

I was surprised to find out that methods of detoxification have been around for almost four thousand years. One of the earliest medical textbooks ever discovered, the Ebers Papyrus, found in the sands of Egypt, shows that physicians of long ago were already using enemas to help the body cleanse itself and fight off disease. In India, Ayurvedic medicine also utilizes detoxification methods, including colon cleansing, to treat many chronic conditions and to prevent illness. But the colon is just one of many channels of elimination. This book will discuss other ways to decrease the burden of this toxic load.

One thing is clear, now is the time to *protect yourself*. Let's start by taking a deeper look at the toxicity we receive from products we put on the largest organ of our body: our skin.

WHAT ARE YOU PUTTING ON YOUR SKIN?

Have you ever stopped to question just what we do each day in the name of self-care and beauty? Until recently, would it ever have entered your mind that the cosmetics you have been using contain chemicals that may be making you sick, drying out your skin, and making you fat? Did it ever dawn on any of us that chemicals entering through the skin are as toxic to our systems as if we had ingested them through our mouths?

Over the years, I've spent a small fortune on the "best" cosmetics money could buy, all promising miracles and smelling fantastic. I've been rubbing creams and lotions all over my body in an attempt to make my skin soft, healthy, and appealing.

Now we have the information. This book explains the toxic burden. Now it's important to understand how toxins enter the bloodstream through the skin. So I've interviewed a number of dermatologic experts.

Commercial creams and lotions, no matter how high-end, contain emulsifiers, most often chemicals that allow oils and water to stay mixed, prevent bacteria from growing, and so on. But even though these products are supposed to hydrate the skin, they actually have the opposite effect!

Learning about the standard of skin care products made me look at my products in a whole new light. I started working with an organic formulator who uses only certified toxic-free ingredients. She told me that our skin is made of mechanisms designed to trap water. When we take a bath or shower, our skin doesn't actually absorb water but rather traps it. The problem with commercial creams is that the same chemicals that alter the natural characteristics of oil and water, allowing them to stay mixed, also break down the natural oils in our skin. This allows water to evaporate from our skin, and it also causes our cells to put up a shield. At a cellular level the same thing takes place—your cells put up shields to protect themselves from these chemicals. So now your cells are closed off and can't eliminate waste or take in nutrition. As a result, the cells die prematurely. We get thinner and thinner skin that feels crepey and develops wrinkles.

The worst emulsifiers of all are PEGs. The full name is polyethylene glycol, which is very seldom written out—who wants to bring attention to this dangerous chemical? Anything that lists a PEG in the ingredients has been ethoxylated, or made with ethylene oxide, a very, very toxic chemical. For commercial cosmetic use, this is the supersecret ingredient. It makes textures we like, but unfortunately at great cost to our health. Ethoxylated chemicals are easy to use and have a shelf life of as much as fifty thousand years. (Cosmetics companies really don't have a clue, do they?) Almost all ethoxylated chemicals contain trace amounts of 1, 4-dioxane, which can damage the liver and kidneys and may cause cancer.

The point of this book is that carrying around a toxic burden is a huge component in your inability to shed the pounds, but most people have no idea of the extent of the chemical exposure we are getting from lotions and creams.

PEGs impact the hormonal system and the brain and create a toxic burden in the body. They may cause memory loss. And the big "E" in cosmetics happens in other words like MEA, DEA, TEA, or triethanolamine.

The *E* is for the ethoxylation process. You can look for *eth* in ingredients, or the capital *E;* for instance in baby shampoo it's laur*eth*. From the moment a baby is born, companies are giving away free baby products in the hospital with laureth in them. The baby is then inundated with harmful chemicals, all because this chemical makes lotions easier to produce. Our pure little babies are no longer pure, even moments after they are born.

Even using products labeled organic is no guarantee that they're toxin free. "Certified organic" only means that a government official has said to the farmer, "For seven years we have been able to verify that you have not used insecticides or pesticides." But that government agency doesn't have anything to do with the guy upstream from him who does use chemicals or whether a farmer or manufacturer uses chemicals to extract elements from organic ingredients. There's not a test to verify that level of purity, but products that are "certified toxic free" can help ensure your safety from such chemicals.

With all the toxicity to which humans are exposed (*bombarded* is probably a better word), it's not difficult to imagine what effect this is going to have on us in the long term. Where is this going? Might it even have an impact on our children's fertility? I realize that is a heavy concept, but not acknowledging the severity of the situation only guarantees that it will get worse. Pay attention to the cosmetics, shampoos, conditioners, and tanning lotions you use. Read the labels. Try to eliminate toxic ingredients by selecting natural products. You will find a list of ingredients to avoid at the back of this book.

WHAT HAVE YOU GOT STORED AWAY?

Fat-stored toxins are a major factor in becoming overweight. And you don't lose toxins just because you have lost weight. You have to lose weight smartly, or you could actually make yourself sicker—and fatter. Dieting without detoxing is one of the best ways to get derailed.

According to Dr. Walter Crinnion in his book *Clean, Green, and Lean,*

"When stored fat is mobilized into your bloodstream, fat-soluble toxins—toxins that dissolve in fat and take up residence there—are also released. This breakdown of fat, known as lipolysis, takes place daily—especially at night when your body goes hours without eating. When you are dieting, exercising or experiencing high stress, your lipolysis rate increases and that means a higher than normal amount of persistent poisons is swimming in your bloodstream along with the fats."

If you are not detoxing simultaneously with dieting, a vicious cycle gets initiated. When you diet and exercise, toxins are released from your fat into the bloodstream. These higher concentrations of toxins make you feel sluggish and sick. So you stop exercising and give in to the cravings. That is why many people on diets start feeling lousy, sometimes with headaches, flu-like symptoms, or mood swings—most a result of the increased presence of toxins. But this is exactly when you have to stay with it to succeed in cleaning out your body and losing weight.

> You have to push through.

Detoxification is not for sissies. When the toxins get released, even if you feel sluggish, you have to continue forward with a firm, full commitment. According to Dr. Crinnion, the only solution is "breaking the toxin recirculation cycle."

Sexy Forever will show you the changes you need to make to your diet and lifestyle in order to lose weight and be healthy.

COMING CLEAN: GETTING STARTED

This is a lifestyle change. It's no longer enough to simply cut out the offending foods; you must combat the toxicity in your body by choosing clean, healthy food that has not been contaminated by chemicals. This is crucial and takes a shift in mind-set. Today's standard diet of refined, enriched, preserved, irradiated, genetically modified, pasteurized, homogenized, hydrogenated, and processed foods doesn't begin to meet our nutritional needs. The body needs proper nutrition for fuel. And it needs to be clean to use that nutrition. So we start with detoxification before anything else.

If you still think you don't have a toxic body, let me point out what Dr. Russell Blaylock once told me: "Depending on your exposure, even if you consume organic food, the chemical onslaught for each of us is akin to taking anywhere from a quarter of a teaspoon of, let's say, rat poison daily." Now how long do you think you are going to stay healthy if you're taking rat poison daily? So let's say goodbye to rat poison, hello to health.

There are many ways to detoxify, and you can get started today. Here's a quick roundup before we go deeper.

In order to detoxify your life and your environment you need to:

- Consume fruits and vegetables that are free of pesticides.

- Eat at home more often so you know the exact quality of your food.

- Use safe vegetable washes to remove toxins, chemicals, and aflatoxins (a type of fungus that can lead to liver cancer).

- Choose grass-fed beef and lamb.

- Consume organic pork and poultry.

- Avoid farm-raised fish and high-mercury fish.

There is more:

- It is essential to maintain a household free of toxic chemicals. Remove any chemicals and toxic household cleaners from your home, or at least limit your exposure to them. Substitute natural cleaning products such as distilled white vinegar, baking soda,

CLEAN UP YOUR LIVER

- Twice a day, just before a meal, drink a cup of warm water with the juice of half a fresh lemon or a tablespoon of apple cider vinegar. This lemon water or vinegar water aids in bile formation, resulting in more efficient fat metabolism.

- Eat protein every day, preferably at every meal. The liver needs the amino acids from protein to produce bile and to make enzymes used in detoxification.

- Eggs are a great source of protein, plus they have the added benefit of being naturally rich in lecithin, a substance your liver needs in order to produce bile.

- Get essential fatty acids daily, especially omegas-3s, from walnuts, flax-seed and/or flaxseed oil, salmon, fish oil supplements, or cod liver oil.

- Essential minerals such as copper, magnesium, and zinc play an important role in liver detoxification, along with vitamin C, most of the B vitamins, folic acid, and flavonoids (found in richly colored vegetables such as sweet red peppers).

These things done on a daily basis will help with liver detoxification, which aids in reducing your toxic burden, thereby allowing you to lose weight.

borax, lemon juice, citrus cleaners, castile soaps, and safe commercial products. These items can be purchased from health food stores or grocery stores like Whole Foods.

- Use certified toxin-free skin and body care products. You don't want to be putting chemicals on your skin when you are trying to detoxify.

- Pay attention to the air you breathe. Install air filters or commit to proper ventilation. The average American spends most of his or her time indoors; the quality of that air becomes crucial. I had not heard of "sick buildings" until I experienced one for myself. Consider air filters that are available for home use. Common household plants can also be used as filters to remove pollution from indoors.

- Filter your water. Unfortunately, our tap water is a major source of toxic chemicals that our overworked livers are required to process. A water filter will help. And reverse osmosis filters are essential if you have fluoride in your water system.

FOODS THAT HEAL, NOT HARM

Eliminate poor food choices: processed foods, diet foods, diet sodas, fast foods. None of these foods have any nutritional value. If it comes in a bag or a box, it is most likely processed and contains chemicals and preservatives. Once you wean yourself from these foods, the cravings will go away. Your body will crave food that provides nutrients. Think of drug addicts—they have to go through a period of detox, which can be very difficult depending on the degree of addiction, but if they get to the other side, they can live the rest of their lives without cravings.

Think real food. Choose clean foods like grass-fed beef and lamb, organic chicken, and natural pork. Choose organic fruits and vegetables. In fact, shop the periphery of the supermarket—that's where you'll find meat, fish, dairy, fruits, and vegetables.

Here's my criterion for choosing food: if you can pick it, pluck it, milk it, or shoot it, you can eat it! Outside of that guideline, you are getting into fake-food land, where nutritional content is absent. If you read labels and find something you can't pronounce, chances are it has been made in a chemical lab.

Beef isn't a problem if it is grass-fed and organic. The naturally occurring fat in grass-fed beef is good for you and aids in healthy cell building, but beef has been demonized. Funnily enough, it was Dr. Frederick Stare of Harvard University, head of the nutrition department for many years, and his study on Irish brothers that positively correlated a high intake of *vegetable oils*, not animal fats, *with heart disease*. Shortly after he became department head, however, the university received several large grants from the *food processing industry*. (You connect the dots.) After that, Dr. Stare's weekly columns began assuring the public there was nothing wrong with white bread, sugar, and highly processed foods! He recommended one cup of *corn oil* (omega-6 bad oil) per day to prevent heart disease and in one article he even recommended Coca-Cola (with high-fructose corn syrup) as a snack! One could make a guess here: Money talks.

Choose cold-water fish such as wild-caught salmon and sardines. Eat only minimal amounts of fish that tend to be high in mercury, such as tuna, swordfish, and halibut. Fish get exposed to mercury from polluted water and by eating smaller fish; they absorb the entire load of mercury that the smaller fish has eaten during its lifetime. In this way the big fish adds the small fish's mercury buildup to its own.

You can also be exposed to mercury through silver amalgam dental fillings, emissions from coal-fired power plants, auto parts, fluorescent light bulbs, medical products, and some over-the-counter products such as topical antiseptics, stimulant laxatives, diaper rash ointment, eyedrops, and nasal sprays. Mercury is very toxic and very slow to leave the body; after consuming mercury-laden fish it can take a whole year to get the blood levels down to a normal range. But that's not all. Mercury's half life (the time it takes for a chemical to be reduced by half) in the brain takes over one year.

I'm not trying to overwhelm you here—all the positive steps you take add up to great health and the healthy weight you want.

YOU CAN'T AFFORD ORGANIC?

Unfortunately, organic food is still more expensive than nonorganic. This creates a quandry for many who can't aford it. Nonorganic food will continue to make you unhealthy and your weight will further spiral out of control. The cost of sickness down the road will surely outweigh the price of organic food today. In time, I believe, with increasing knowledge and demand, the price of organic food will decrease. In fact, people are catching on, and you've probably noticed that organic food is much less expensive than it was, say, a year ago. So that's hopeful.

If you can't afford to buy organic food, perhaps you can create a garden in your yard, or participate in a community farm where everyone is allowed to grow on a small parcel of land approved by the city. Growing your own food is very thrilling. I have my own organic garden, and I choose our meals daily depending on what is of peak ripeness on that particular day. One of the great pleasures of my life is to work with my vegetable garden; it feeds my love of food, love of cooking, love of healthy living, and love of nature, all in one. In today's hectic world, planting a garden might be the one thing that pulls you back into a simpler time, a purer time, a calmer time . . . just something to think about.

If you simply can't afford organic food and you can't grow your own, there is a solution. It's crucial to wash nonorganic foods carefully to cut down on ingested toxins. Soak all nonorganic food for twenty minutes in water to which you've added salt and fresh lemon juice or vinegar, or purchase a good vegetable wash to remove the toxins as best you can.

Certain foods in the produce section tend to be very high in pesticides. If you can't buy these organic or avoid them then follow the washing instructions to make them less toxic.

Fruits and Vegetables Highest in Pesticides

Grapes	Peaches
Lettuce	Strawberries
Apples	Pears
Bell peppers	Kale
Carrots	Celery
Nectarines	

Fruits and Vegetables Lowest in Pesticides

Broccoli	Papayas
Bananas	Mangoes
Avocados	Pineapples
Cabbage	Onions
Watermelon	Shallots
Sweet peas	Kiwis
Sweet corn	Asparagus

Even though these are all yummy and nutritious foods and are the *least* contaminated, be sure to wash them well, as they are not free of toxins. To reduce toxic exposure before eating nonorganic pears, nectarines, and potatoes, soak them in a bowl of vinegar (approximately 4 tablespoons) and enough water to cover, then peel them before eating.

Soak vegetables like bell peppers and celery in a bowl of water with the juice of a fresh lemon for twenty minutes, then scrub with a vegetable brush. Soak cherries in this lemon water for sixty minutes.

There are two nonorganic fruits you really should never eat: apples and grapes. A toxic pesticide called cryolite goes through the skin of these fruits and permeates them entirely. But the organic versions of grapes and apples are loaded with incredible nutrients and enzymes, so if you can swing it, go organic here.

Unfortunately, poison-sprayed food that has not been thoroughly washed is so toxic that the chemicals outweigh the good the food could do in its natural state. As you know, without sufficient nutrients the brain keeps signaling the body to want more and more food. These cravings are usually for sugar or carbohydrates, since these are the quickest sources of energy. Don't be hard on yourself. It's not about your will at this point; there are physical needs for these foods, as harmful as they may be. But over time these cravings will go away.

AROUND THE HOUSE

We already talked about this at the beginning of the chapter, so I won't go into detail here. Just go green for all household products. The commercial cleaners and chemicals you have been using liberally all these years make your home toxic and may be linked to many conditions including autoimmune diseases and allergies. Green and natural household cleaners are now available everywhere, both in stores and online. This simple change is another valuable step in detoxifying your body.

Then switch to chemical-free cosmetics. Everything you put on your skin goes into your bloodstream. What is the sense of eating organic food and getting rid of household chemicals, and then loading up on chemicals on your skin?

GET HEALTHY, STAY SEXY

GOING THE EXTRA MILE

These simple changes I've described above will help. You'll feel energized, your appetite will diminish, bloating will subside, and your weight will start to drop. I've got some more in my bag of tricks, if you're willing to go a little deeper. Stay with me!

Get the Patch

I am ambassador for a company called LifeWave, which has developed amazing nanotechnology patches that help your body produce glutathione, a key component in your body's natural detoxification mechanism. Glutathione is an antioxidant that protects our cells from damage by free radicals and holds off the ravages of aging (including weight gain). We stop making glutathione around age forty, which is why our bodies become less resistant to disease and less able to fight off the toxins we all encounter in our everyday lives. By wearing one of these patches daily, you clean out toxins from your cells. At night I wear a patch to help my body produce carnosine, an antioxidant that repairs cell damage from free radicals.

These patches are a simple way to fight the chemical onslaught. Wearing the glutathione patch can help greatly in detoxing your body. It's very simple—you wear the patch three fingers below your navel and change it every day. Along with good nutrition and eliminating outside chemicals as best you can, you will be well on your way to good health and a thin body. (See Resources for more information.)

Consider Colonics

Colonic irrigation is one of the least expensive, most effective ways to cleanse the large intestine of accumulated toxins and waste products. Colonics draw toxins from the blood and lymph back into the colon for excretion. Colonic irrigation lasts thirty-five to forty minutes and cleans the entire five feet of the colon, unlike an enema, which cleanses only the lower eight to twelve inches of the bowel. Enemas are a good way of detoxing the lower bowel, particularly lukewarm coffee enemas that are not too strong.

Take an Infrared Sauna

This is a highly effective, but very expensive, way to detoxify. The body uses its own internally generated heat to protect itself from viruses, bacteria, and other harmful substances—a fever is the body's attempt to destroy invading organisms and to sweat out impurities through the skin.

An infrared sauna has heat levels that are generally kept around 140°F. The heat stress removes calcium deposits from the blood vessels and breaks down scar tissue from blood vessel walls. Some studies demonstrate that saunas can remove chemicals such as DDE, PCBs, and dioxin from fat cells.

Home units are available for purchase for $1,200; again, this is very expensive, but I want you to know all your options. I take a forty-five-minute sauna two or three times a week, and I am always sure to drink lots of water before and after to get maximum benefits. Of course, as with any measure affecting your health, before you try a treatment, consult with a doctor or knowledgeable and experienced expert.

Consider Chelation Therapy

Chelation therapy draws lead, mercury, and other heavy metals out of the body. Chelation refers to a method of binding up toxins such as heavy metals and bodily wastes and removing them, while at the same time increasing blood flow. In chelation therapy a substance called EDTA is administered intravenously and binds to various toxic metals in the blood such as mercury, lead, cadmium, and aluminum. The toxins are then flushed from the body through the kidneys. EDTA is three times *less* toxic than aspirin and has been tested and used safely for the past thirty years on an estimated half million patients, including me. Other detoxification methods use ultraviolet light or hydrogen peroxide. Your antiaging doctor will be familiar with this process, and you can discuss with him or her which treatment would be best for you.

Get a Lymph Massage

The lymphatic system is a complicated network of vessels, ducts, and nodes that moves fluid between the cells and tissues and produces and distributes the infection-fighting and scavenging cells of the body. It feeds literally every tissue and organ and the blood. It is the transportation highway for the immune and repair functions of the body. When the lymph system is functioning properly it effectively cleanses the tissues, aids in cellular repair, and eliminates toxins.

When the lymph system becomes congested, it deprives the cells of oxygen and affects the ability of the body to rid itself of its own waste material. Over time, other body systems that rely on the lymphatic system for waste removal will become compromised, setting the stage for pain and disease. A sure sign of lymph congestion is sore or swollen lymph glands, which are most noticeable in the neck, armpits, and groin. Illnesses ranging from allergies to fibrocystic disease and even cancer can be related to lymph congestion.

Correct diet, infrared saunas, and manual lymphatic massage can prevent or reverse lymph congestion and will stimulate the flow of the lymph. I work with Cynthia Story, a certified lymphatic specialist in Montecito, California. If you're considering this treatment, be sure to choose an experienced therapist. Someone who isn't can actually aggravate a patient's condition.

Because of the time-consuming nature of lymph massage, a lot of doctors are turning to a noninvasive handheld instrument known as the light beam generator (LBG) to restore lymph function and eliminate wastes. This machine penetrates many times deeper than lymphatic massage alone and also increases the effectiveness of manual drainage of the lymph system. See if your doctor will purchase one for office use; it can't hurt to ask.

Try an Ondamed Machine

This is a very sophisticated piece of equipment you should urge your doctor to buy. It is a cellular-electrical-biofeedback machine used for acute pain management and lymphatic congestion, among other things. This machine has been used successfully since 1993. It releases a "spectrum of low-level pulsing magnetic fields that induce the flow of microcurrents within the tissues"—which in English means it is able to locate underlying dysfunction and provide treatment for the patient. It promotes improved circulation, wound healing, bone regrowth, and pain relief for conditions such as fibromyalgia. (Go to SuzanneSomers.com for a list of Ondamed practitioners.)

Get Oxygenated

Hyperbaric oxygen is often used by cancer patients to successfully detoxify after chemotherapy. This is an expensive treatment and involves breathing high concentrations of oxygen in a pressurized chamber.

RELEASE YOUR TOXIC BURDEN FOREVER

Whether you make small changes or large changes, one by one you can start to eliminate toxins from your life. You don't have to do it all at once, but with each step you are closer to significantly lowering your own personal toxic burden. Each change will add to the quality of your health and life, and I promise you will feel an inner peace that you are reducing your exposure to chemicals.

Cancer was a major wake-up call for me and forced me to examine my lifestyle and dietary habits. I was lucky to have taken charge of the disease with a firm resolve to eat as though my life depended on it, which it did. Cleaning out my house and medicine cabinet of chemical cosmetics and household cleaners was the next logical step.

> Every step we take to eliminate chemicals from our
> lives is a step toward health and looking good.

As I cleaned up my life and cleaned out my body I lost weight. Those extra menopausal pounds that had plagued me for years, especially around the tops of my hips and abdomen—the pounds that for the first time didn't respond to my Somersize way of life—miraculously seemed to dissolve. I got back to 127 pounds—my perfect weight! That's when I began making the connection between balanced hormones, eating clean food, avoiding chemicals, healing my gut, and taking proper supplementation.

You don't have to go cold turkey. Of course, the faster you want the weight to go away, the more changes you will have to make. But this is a program for life. A new way of life—one where you are committed to living a long, healthy life up until the very last breath. What a beautiful thought.

When you change the way you eat, when you change the way you live your life, when you switch your household cleaners to natural products, your health will get better. When you are healthy, losing weight is easier.

This is your choice to make. That choice determines whether your health will soar or spiral downward, and it determines whether you will gain control of your weight forever or continue to yo-yo for the rest of your life.

It's up to you—by making simple changes you can restore your energy, good health, and slim body.

BALANCE YOUR HORMONES

Dr. Jonathan Wright is called the father of bioidentical hormones because he was the first physician to prescribe them in the United States twenty-five years ago. He teaches other doctors the art of individualizing natural hormones and has been one of my greatest teachers. According to Dr. Wright, "Diet and exercise are always of primary importance, but a little-known fact is that it is easier to control and lose weight if bioidentical hormones are used. This applies to perimenopausal women, menopausal women, and andropausal men. Replacing hormones with real, natural bioidentical hormones reduces our risk of cognitive decline (foggy brain), heart disease, and Alzheimer's. Bioidentical hormones also help maintain women's lung function, control weight, and restore sexuality."

Sounds pretty great, doesn't it? Isn't this what we all want?

I am living proof that it is achievable. With balanced hormones and my detoxed body, weight is no longer an issue, but if I get lax and allow myself to be overly exposed to chemicals and eat badly, or ignore my newly found food intolerances to eggs and yeast (sigh), I gain it back in the wrong places. (I'll tell you a little more about that later in this chapter. When I hit forty, I experienced much of what I suspect you may be going through right now.)

Now I never let my hormones become imbalanced. Without balance I feel awful, and that includes bloating and lethargy. I am not a thin person in a supermodel-type body. I am rounder (those big breasts) and I have small hips. But I have had trouble keeping my waist at the trim desirable size I once was in my *Three's Company* days.

I often speak of aging as aspirational, meaning that you can achieve optimal health by maintaining perfect hormonal balance, regardless of the chronological clock. It is very difficult for women and men to wade through all the untruths, myths, and lack of understanding relative to hormone replacement. For example, the most widely used estrogen replacement, Premarin, is made from pregnant mare's urine. Why would we want to take horse estrogen? Instead, bioidentical hormones (biologically identical to the human hormone, an exact replica of what our bodies make or made) are the perfect answer. I have been restoring my lost hormones with bioidenticals for almost fifteen years. I believe that it has arrested the aging process for me dramatically.

I had three years of agony that no one seemed to understand. "It can't be menopause," I thought; "I'm only forty! But it sure *seems* like my thighs are growing." When I was a kid, I was always the skinny one—people called me Bony Mahoney (Mahoney being my maiden name) or Beanpole. I was so skinny I was embarrassed to be seen in a bathing suit. The boys made fun of me, saying I was "flat as a pancake." I grew out of that, but when I reached my fortieth year, suddenly I was struggling to button my pants and self-conscious about my growing waistline.

What happened? Two things: the changing toxic planet coupled with declining hormones. A lethal combination if you are trying to stay thin.

Hormones! Declines in levels of hormones start early now, often in the mid- to late thirties, with some lucky ones making it to their forties intact. But eventually we all get there. Come to think of it, once I hit my forties I wasn't very interested in sex either. When did that happen? I had always loved it!

But did I make the connection? Noooooo! I suffered through another ten years before I understood, and during three of those years life would be a living hell due to dramatic symptoms of declining hormones. I remember saying to my husband one day that my clothes were shrinking.

LET'S TALK ABOUT SEX

It's not over just because you have hit middle age. Not at all! I talk about sex because a healthy person is a sexual person. You will not feel sexual if you are not hormonally balanced, and an imbalanced person is not healthy. It's important to work at achieving hormonal balance. Feeling "in the mood" will be a good indicator that all is well again.

At middle age a woman's sex hormones—estrogen, progesterone, and testosterone—start to decline. The more these hormones decline, the less interested she becomes in sex. When these hormones completely drain out, that's when you hear women say things like, "Oh, I'm past that." Not a good sign. It's an indicator that decline and deterioration have begun. It's all downhill from there. The medications begin (and in the western medical world they have a pill for everything—although did you ever notice that there is no Viagra for women?). The perfect way to restore your sexuality is to balance your hormones.

Ha! I was now two sizes bigger, but I hadn't changed the size clothing I was buying. I would delude myself into thinking I was just bloated and that when it went away the outfit would fit. Denial! And I got good at hiding it. If I had to appear on TV I would literally starve myself for a couple of weeks to slim down, but this kind of weight loss is always temporary and confuses your body. Missing meals makes you fat because the body readjusts to expect less food. When you go back to normal eating the body doesn't know what to do with this extra food, so it stores it as fat.

My life is not about deprivation. I enjoy delicious meals with healthy fats, I eat until I am full and satisfied, and I remain thin. I enjoy a robust sex life. I sleep eight hours nightly. And while I avoid chemicals in my home and eat organic food, none of this good feeling would be possible without natural bioidentical hormone replacement.

Hormones are the juice of youth. Hormones are a language instructing the body to feel good, have energy, and be healthy and sexual. Hormones regulate our body heat and our ability to think and feel good; hormones keep our bones strong, our brain sharp, and our organs functioning. Hormones are what give us our good health, and the symptoms we associate with aging are often simply related to this decline in hormones. That is why menopausal women experience hot flashes, sleepless nights, tremendous weight gain, and a loss of libido. Without enough sex hormones you can't feel sexy.

When it comes to aging, the only choices are to accept *deterioration* or to choose *restoration*. I have chosen restoration. What does that mean? First of all, I recognized that I needed to restore all of my hormones to optimal levels.

In this chapter, with the help of Dr. Jonathan Wright, I briefly explain how the hormonal system works and why imbalanced or declining hormones lead to weight gain and feeling like you are no longer the person you used to be.

It's important to understand that hormones are like a symphony that requires all the instruments to be in tune in order to be *harmonic*. Stress disrupts this harmony and causes changes in your hormones. It makes your body out of tune, then your adrenals go on high alert, which starts a cascade of hormonal imbalances, and symptoms then begin to occur. Over time stress and hormone changes cause hot flashes, weight gain, and an inability to sleep.

Stress and toxicity blunt hormone production. This is why younger and younger women are experiencing hormonal decline.

The problem is the way our high-stress lifestyles affect our adrenal glands. The adrenals, in simple terms, produce the stress hormones adrenaline and cortisol, whose job is to rev up the body when needed. In paleolithic times this would be when being chased by a saber-toothed tiger, but in today's world we live the equivalent of being chased by that tiger all the time. Our adrenals are on overload. When this happens, a cascade of bodily problems begins.

High adrenal outputs can cause dizziness, which usually sends people to the nearest neurologist. I have seen girlfriends go through this over and over again. I always tell them, "Before you agree to all those expensive tests, why don't you do a twenty-four-hour urine test and check your adrenal levels and all your other hormones?" When high adrenal output is evident from a twenty-four-hour urine test, the next thing to do is to look at the levels of progesterone and estrogen. Most likely they will be in decline, and restoring those to optimal levels usually balances out the adrenals. If you flatline your adrenals from extreme stress (overwork, death, divorce, financial upheaval), then natural bioidentical cortisol (hydrocortisone) may be required.

This is why I stress that starting from age forty you should obtain the services of a qualified antiaging doctor (go to SuzanneSomers.com), one who is current on the effects of declining hormones. Most often, though, declining hormones and the resulting symptoms are not understood by your regular doctor, who may order a battery of expensive tests and unnecessary CAT scans. (CAT scans carry with them large amounts of radiation, which is carcinogenic. Recently a report came out saying that CAT scans carry many times more radiation than originally thought. Remember, all toxicity is a route to weight gain and disease, and unnecessary radiation is just another toxin.) How many times has a woman been diagnosed incorrectly with a neurologic or autoimmune disease like lupus, MS, or fibromyalgia when she was simply hormonally imbalanced?

Conventional medical treatment of these symptoms requires huge amounts of toxic pharmaceutical drugs, which cause side effects requiring more drugs . . . raising cortisol levels further. High cortisol makes sleeping impossible (you're running from the tiger, remember?), so now you need toxic sleeping pills. This inability to sleep raises production of the stress hormone cortisol, and when cortisol levels go up, your blood sugar increases, making it difficult to burn stored body fat.

When cortisol and insulin levels are off, the thyroid (the gland that produces the fat-burning hormone) acts up and lowers the energy in the body. Hormones produced by the thyroid regulate cells and organs by stimulating the mitochondria, the cells' little powerhouses.

When the thyroid gland works correctly, it warms the body, stimulates energy by freeing heat and energy, and prevents sensitivity to hot and cold (especially in the extremities). Thyroid also stimulates fat burning, helps dissolve cholesterol, and makes the arterial walls more supple, thereby opening the arteries and moderating blood pressure. The symptoms of a low thyroid are pretty easy to spot: dry skin, constipation, stiff joints, sensitivity to heat and cold, and fatigue—you feel very tired . . . exhausted.

As I've noted, this cascade of symptoms is often a result of declining hormones, starting with estrogen and progesterone. Estrogen and progesterone are the minor hormones, but why they are called minor makes little sense because when these molecules get out of balance life becomes very, very difficult. Nothing minor about it. I call this imbalance the Seven Dwarves of Menopause: Itchy, Bitchy, Sleepy, Sweaty, Bloated, Forgetful, and All Dried Up!

There are three well-known components to what we understand as estrogen:

- Estriol (cancer protective)

- Estradiol (pro-carcinogenic)

- Estrone (pro-carcinogenic)

This is why there is much confusion about estrogen replacement causing breast cancer. Even conventional doctors now acknowledge that horse-urine-derived estrogen (Premarin) increases risk of cancer and other diseases. The carcinogenic effect is worse when a synthetic progestin (like Provera) is combined with estrogen. That is why so many women got breast cancer and estrogen got a bad rap. It was never made clear that the study was done on horse hormones like Premarin, not on hormones identical to those produced in the human body. There has not been a single reported case of cancer as a result of bioidentical hormones.

Women using natural-to-the-human-body estrogens should also use natural progesterone (not synthetic progestin) and follow other steps to reduce cancer risk such as ensuring optimal vitamin D status. This usually requires supplementation with at least 5,000 IU of vitamin D each day— far more than is found in conventional multinutrient products.

Natural progesterone opposes the cell-proliferating impact of estrogen on female reproductive organs. In our younger years, we naturally produced abundant amounts of progesterone two weeks out of every month.

Menopause unfortunately results in the rapid decline of production of natural progesterone. So when doctors prescribe estrogen without natural progesterone, they are creating an imbalance whereby there is not enough natural progesterone to oppose the estrogen drugs they are prescribing. Remember that the drug they too often prescribed contained Provera, which is not natural progesterone and has in fact been linked to numerous health problems. But when estrogen is *opposed* with progesterone two weeks of every month (like we used to make when we were having a period), we are more protected from getting cancer. When estrogen and progesterone are replaced with bioidenticals in normal physiologic levels in the right ratios, individualized for each person, the effect is amazing.

My doctor keeps track of my estrogen levels with urine and blood tests once or twice a year. He checks for balance not only in the ratio of estrogen and progesterone but also in these three well-known components and all the minor components that make up what we know as estrogen. Through testing, my doctor (Jonathan Wright) was able to determine that my body does not make the usual amount of the essential component of estrogen known as estriol. This is a major factor because estriol is a very important cancer-protective part of estrogen. Without it a woman is set up for cancer. There is no defense. I am one of those women. Lucky for me, Dr. Wright was able to figure this out and very likely has prevented me from a recurrence. Along with my bioidentical estradiol, he prescribes the right dosage of daily estriol.

I am certain that a huge contributing factor in why I got breast cancer was a lack of estriol in my body (along with twenty-two years of so-called safe birth control pills). I see estriol, which sits at the estrogen receptor site (guarding against too much pro-carcinogenic estrogen), as a little ninja warrior protecting me.

When your levels of estrogen and progesterone begin to decline, imbalances may arise in other hormones: thyroid, insulin, adrenals, and cortisol. Imagine a teeter-totter: when one hormone drops other hormones rise. Imbalanced hormones lead to weight gain. You see it all the time, and until you understand this you will be in a constant battle with your weight and the symptoms of hormonal decline.

What the body wants is "just right," like Goldilocks—not too much, not too little. For instance, if you don't have enough estrogen or progesterone you will experience bloating and other symptoms. If you have too much estrogen or progesterone, you will experience bloating and other symptoms including weight gain. Just-right levels of hormones create optimal health, but when those levels aren't right we can get symptoms big-time; depression, sleeplessness, foggy thinking, brittle bones, heart disease, and high blood pressure are all part of the signs of imbalance. Conventional medicine most often treats these symptoms with an array of drugs: for depression, Prozac; inability to sleep, Ambien or Lunesta; foggy thinking, Alzheimer's medications; brittle bones, Fosamax; heart weakness, Lipitor (a dreadful dangerous drug; see the chapter on statins in my book *Breakthrough*). Add to this the caffeine and alcohol women are consuming to get up and then to come down and you can see why the present template of aging is a long, slow march to the nursing home; that is, if their overweight bodies don't do them in first.

What a crappy way to enter midlife! With hormones restored, life gets better and better and you get thinner.

Hormones are not understood by most conventional doctors. At present in our medical schools, our doctors receive only four hours of instruction in prescribing hormones, which is why it is essential to work with a doctor who has chosen to specialize in bioidentical hormone replacement. You can find the right doctor by going to SuzanneSomers.com and clicking on Doctor Resource Guide. You will find one nearest you.

LOSE WEIGHT BY BALANCING YOUR HORMONES

Hormonal health is the key to losing weight; you can't do it any other way. Dr. Wright explains in this next section why you are getting fat as a result of hormonal imbalance.

It is also important to understand that men have hormones that become

REMEMBER PMS?

Premenstrual syndrome results from the dipping and falling of estrogen right before your period when the progesterone is not rising quickly enough. A similar type of hormone imbalance occurs during perimenopause, a very undertreated phase of initial hormonal decline. During perimenopause, estrogen and progesterone are dipping and surging out of control, and they trigger the brain that we are about to be no longer reproductive. Biologically speaking we are only here for one reason: perpetuation of the species. When the brain perceives us to be nonreproductive, its job is to eliminate us. Nature wants to make way for the healthy reproductive ones—perpetuation of the species. As hormones diminish, the body tries to compensate for the loss. It fattens up to protect our now brittle bones from lack of estrogen and progesterone, our brain loses its edge (a lack of estrogen getting to the brain can trigger migraine headaches and foggy thinking). Then our cortisol goes so high we can't sleep. Chronic high stress hormones can lead to heart attack or stroke (the leading killer of women . . . hmm, chicken or egg?). All these symptoms are a result of declining and imbalanced hormones.

imbalanced due to the aging process or stress. When men decline hormonally they begin to fall apart just like women. Couple this with the chemical onslaught of everyday life and the result is disastrous: men gain weight, their skin sags, their guts become compromised, they develop food intolerances, they don't sleep well, and they lose their sex drive. But it all happens gradually, so no one really pays attention until the symptoms appear. And then it is not pretty. Men, too, get sick as a result of hormonal decline. Cancer, diabetes, heart disease, and Alzheimer's are rampant among men.

Let's hear what Dr. Jonathan Wright says about this issue:

Let's examine each hormone and its effects on weight gain. Balance is what is desired. Balanced hormones make weight loss possible; without balance you are climbing uphill.

DHEA. DHEA is another important hormone to understand, especially in relation to belly fat. In an article published in the *Journal of the American Medical Association* in 2004, a double-blind study showed that people taking a DHEA supplement lost two pounds, while a placebo group gained one pound, which is not an impressive difference. But the women in the DHEA group lost 10 percent of their abdominal fat (this was tested through an MRI study) and the men in the DHEA group lost 7 percent of their abdominal fat.

There is a strong benefit regarding metabolic syndrome (a precursor to type 2 diabetes), which is a condition of insulin resistance, high cholesterol and high triglyciderides, high blood pressure, and obesity (especially abdominal). Multiple studies show that DHEA reduces insulin resistance. DHEA also has great value for people who have already progressed to type 2 diabetes. DHEA helps transform cortisol (the active, weight-increasing form) back into cortisone. And the DHEA speeds cortisol inactivation (bringing it down, which is a good thing).

Progesterone. This is a vital hormone known to have thermogenic (heat- and temperature-increasing, fat-burning) effects. When a woman has a progesterone surge (a normal part of her menstrual cycle), it causes the body temperature to rise at midnight. An ovulating woman's body temperature remains higher during the second half of her menstrual cycle. Higher body temperature means slightly more energy burned (this is good if you want to lose weight). There are no studies at present on bio-identical progesterone and weight loss, but it is highly probable that bioidentical progesterone, when studied, will be found to help in weight loss.

Testosterone. Testosterone is an important hormone for many reasons. It decreases abdominal fat and builds muscle in many older men.

In some people, it also improves insulin sensitivity and improves blood sugar control. But there is one hazard: as many as one-third of men who use supplemental testosterone also make excess estrogen from testosterone itself, a condition called hyperaromatization. This works against weight loss, and in some cases causes weight gain. Plus, it is dangerous for the prostate gland. Careful testing will usually reveal insulin resistance, a forerunner of type 2 diabetes. This is all completely reversible with diet, exercise, and proper supplementation.

Human growth hormone. HGH is a very misunderstood hormone. It gets a bad rap in the media from those who usually have no comprehension of the incredible benefits of supplementation in proper dosages. Instead, they report on athletes who may take a hundred times more than physiologically required, which *is* dangerous to the body.

Human growth hormone is something we all make in our own bodies, even as adults. If HGH levels are low or low normal then raising them to within the normal adult range helps reduce fat and increase muscle, and is very unlikely to be harmful. Testosterone, DHEA, and thyroid (and probably estrogen) all stimulate the internal production of HGH. Estrogen also regulates growth hormone use in the body.

HGH itself is injectable and expensive. Substances that stimulate the body's production of HGH are available in oral or injectible forms and are less expensive. HCG (human chorionic gonadotropin; see next section) also stimulates HGH production.

Human chorionic gonadotropin. HCG suppresses your appetite by causing low-level nausea (the nausea associated with pregnancy is believed to be due to the surge of HCG during pregnancy). Some practitioners claim HCG is an effective weight loss tool, but success requires severe calorie restriction (fewer than 500 calories per day). HCG is injected but much less expensive than HGH. HCG can stimulate production of testosterone, especially if LH (luteinizing hormone) levels are also low.

Insulin. Insulin is the fat-storing hormone. High levels of insulin lead to weight gain. Insulin production is overstimulated by consumption of sugar and carbohydrates, especially refined carbohydrates. This is a special problem for individuals from families with a predisposition to type 2 diabetes. In men, high insulin levels are also very bad for the cardiovascular system and prostate gland. DHEA and testosterone (along with vitamin D, omega-3 fatty acids, chromium, biotin, and many other nutrients and botanicals, especially the natural plant alkaloid berberine) lower insulin resistance and therefore insulin levels for both men and women. With women the decline in estrogen and progesterone shoots insulin levels high. (Remember the teeter-totter?) As the minor hormones (estrogen, progesterone, and testosterone) dip, the gender-neutral hormones (insulin, thyroid, adrenals, and cortisol) rise.

So for women, by allowing your estrogen, progesterone, and testosterone levels to decline, you set yourself up for weight gain from high insulin and cortisol. In addition, you no longer have the fat-burning benefits of a properly working thyroid. And your adrenals are high (cortisol again), so now you can't sleep, and are putting yourself at risk for a heart attack. This entire cascade is due to declining estrogen, progesterone, and DHEA (which declines in both sexes starting at age thirty to thirty-five, allowing cortisol to start a slow upward creep well before menopause). So you can see that all the hormones are affected when one is off. When your doctor says you have high insulin levels, take the information seriously. (You may need to check with a doctor who knows how to do proper insulin resistance testing with a sugar challenge to get this information, though.)

Cortisol. High cortisol levels make sleep impossible. On the other hand, if your cortisol is low, weight is lost in excess (but this is unhealthy weight loss). If cortisol is overactive (high), either systemically or intracellularly (in fat cells), it promotes weight gain.

When estrogen drops, cortisol rises, because the inhibiting effect estrogen had on the enzyme that transforms cortisone into active cortisol is now mostly gone.

High cortisol can be rectified by estrogen, DHEA, and testosterone supplementation in a bioidentical form. Because high cortisol promotes the formation of new fat cells from connective tissue cells, you want to get that down, and can do so by replacing the hormones that have declined with age.

Thyroid. Thyroid is the fat-burning hormone. If thyroid levels are low, thyroid supplementation can promote weight loss. Blood tests frequently miss weak thyroid function, and doctors often don't even check rT3 (reverse T3) levels, so it is important that you find a doctor who does not rely solely on lab results and will conduct a thorough clinical evaluation. And you need a doctor who understands how to read the overly broad ranges of normal, an example being the "shrinking TSH range." If you're scratching your head, let me explain.

Kathy Simpson wrote in her book *The Woman's Guide to Thyroid Health*: "With hypothyroidism [low thyroid], we don't metabolize food effectively and the calories we consume turn into fat instead of energy. This weight gain is insidious, and neither diet nor exercise resolves it. When weight gain is caused strictly by low thyroid function and not other endocrine deficiencies as well, fat tends to be symmetrically distributed on the body. . . . When low pituitary function is at the root of low thyroid function, weight gain is generally confined to the area from your abdomen to just above your knees. The skin of a person with hypothyroidism also takes on a flabby look, as overall musculature is affected, too."

Symptoms of an underactive thyroid can include yellow palms, yellow bottoms of feet, missing the outer third of the eyebrows, constipation, slow pulse, cold hands, frequent infections, sensitivity to heat and cold, reduced sweating, dry skin, tongue swelling, and others. You don't need to have all of these symptoms for thyroid to be a factor. Any one of these can be an indicator of low thyroid.

Constipation is extremely common with low thyroid. Both digestion of food and excretion of wastes are slowed along with everything else in the body. The specific cause is deficient muscular action of the abdominal walls and intestines. Bowel movements should occur every twelve to twenty-four hours, but if your thyroid is low they may occur much less frequently, in some cases just once a week. This results in painful hemorrhoids and painful bowel movements, and causes a buildup of toxins because waste products are not excreted as they should be. The fermentation of wastes caused by the extended time it takes for food to move through your digestive tract often results in a lot of gas, which further distends your abdomen.

> Imbalanced hormones can cause mild to severe
> bloating. Thyroid, if low, could be your culprit.

Many environmental chemicals have structures very similar to certain hormones and are toxic to the thyroid. These chemicals can fit into the cellular receptors for these thyroid hormones, with serious consequences. Many of these chemicals mimic estrogen, but some also interfere with the usage and metabolism of thyroid, testosterone, and other hormones. When thyroid function is affected by these chemicals, it can't do its job of destroying poisonous substances and infectious agents. Dr. Davis Lamson, a colleague of mine at Tahoma Clinic, has shown that toxic metals such as lead, mercury, cadmium, and many others can cause elevations of the "blocking" thyroid hormone, reverse T3 or rT3. A chelation test will measure metal toxicity to determine if this is your issue.

Fluoride, heavy metals, chemicals like perchlorates (found in drinking water), and X-rays all can negatively affect the thyroid. Also, certain medications damage or suppress thyroid function, including lithium (at prescription doses), birth control pills, beta-blockers, phenytoin, theophylline, antacids that contain aluminum, sulfa drugs, antihistamines, and chemotherapy drugs. Imbalances of estrogen and progesterone can suppress the thyroid, too.

For more information on BHRT, see the brief guide at the back of the book, as well as a list of doctors at SuzanneSomers.com.

TO WOMEN WHO HAVE HAD A
HYSTERECTOMY

If you've had a hysterectomy, you must find a doctor who understands the importance of replacing progesterone along with estrogen. Taking estrogen without natural progesterone creates imbalances in the body that can lead to cancer and unwanted weight gain. Estrogen and progesterone should be replaced in a cyclical manner, mimicking nature. The prevailing thought of most doctors is that after a hysterectomy women no longer need progesterone because they do not have a uterus. But this ignores the biological reality that whenever we have estrogen in our bodies we must have progesterone taken cyclically to balance it or our entire endocrine system can be thrown off. Balancing your hormones correctly, even if you have had a hysterectomy, will return your metabolism to normal, and (provided you detoxify and eat properly) you can regain your perfect weight.

When your thyroid is working as it should, you're more able to withstand massive assaults from our environment. And it will assist in ridding your body of its toxic burden, and in turn will have a positive impact on your ability to lose weight.

The incredible impact of replacing declining hormones is that you get to feel like you did when you were young, when weight wasn't difficult to take off. Why was being thin so easy when you were young? You had *balanced hormones*! The difference between then and now is the imbalance.

To rectify the matter, you need to go to a qualified doctor who specializes in bioidentical hormone replacement.

> Working with a doctor who has not specialized in
> bioidentical hormone replacement is like going to a
> plumber for a heart bypass.

Before you go, it makes sense to have your blood tested for essential hormones ahead of time, so the doctor can accurately and immediately prescribe bioidentical hormone replacement that's right for you. To conveniently have your blood tested, log on to SuzanneSomers.com and click on Life Extension. They have a nationwide network that enables people to have their blood conveniently drawn without the need for an appointment. Life Extension's prices are far more reasonable than what commercial laboratories charge. And if you'd like to dig further into this topic, please grab a copy of *Breakthrough* or *Ageless,* as in those books I delve into the entire subject.

STAYING WELL

I take great pains (and I have had the patience) to find and keep hormonal balance. If I can do it, so can you. The effect of balance on my life is fantastic. Every day is a good one and as a result of my choices I am healthy, I'm thin, I have energy, and I feel involved and vital. Plus as an added bonus I have the benefits of youthful hormonal protection against cancer—a win-win.

You have a choice: you can continue to deteriorate, continue to eat an unhealthy diet, continue to surround yourself with chemicals, continue to eat chemicals, continue to take unneeded over-the-counter or prescription drugs, or you can choose health and *change your life!*

Now that you understand how important a role hormones play in the body, you can see that as we age, having a doctor who can help us keep an eye on these systems is very important. If you don't take hormones seriously, what do you expect will happen? Hormonal imbalance leads to weight gain and poor health. Fat is a language. Fat is your body talking, screaming, to be heard. Tell yourself the truth. Stand naked in front of the mirror. Do you like what you see? Do you want to lose weight? Do you want optimal health? Balancing your hormones is a big part of the answer to health and to the weight that just doesn't seem to want to come off. Once your hormones are balanced, the battle will become easier. Without balanced hormones you are fighting a losing battle.

Again, it's a choice: deterioration or restoration!

Choose health and balance, and weight loss will follow!

It's a new concept to go to the doctor when you are well, but as a result of my doing this, I am never sick. I don't remember my last cold or flu, or ache or pain. Not since breast cancer ten years ago, when I changed my whole approach to my health, have I been sick. (There was one exception: during a poisoning that put me in the hospital, as I explained in my last book, *Knockout*.) I have made a commitment to wellness and optimal health and I have never looked back.

As mentioned, to further understand the hormonal system and hormone replacement, I urge you to read my books *Ageless* and *Breakthrough*. If you want a little refresher, see "A Brief Guide to Bioidentical Hormone Replacement" (page 309).

LOSE WEIGHT BY SLEEPING

Every time I give a lecture, the first thing I do is ask for a show of hands, "How many in this room sleep five hours or less?" Inevitably nearly every hand in the room is raised. It seems like no one is sleeping these days, and the big winners are the pharmaceutical companies who continue to come up with sleeping pills that appear to take care of this problem. Unfortunately sleep induced by sleeping pills is not real sleep. It is a suspended state and none of the natural healing work nature has meant to take place during sleep can happen. Sleep is essential for health and sleep controls appetite.

You ask, What does sleep have to do with losing weight? If you don't sleep, losing weight becomes a losing battle and it all has to do with your hormones, especially the very important hormone cortisol. When you reach midlife, as we've discussed, your hormones estrogen and progesterone begin to plummet. As these hormones fall, your cortisol rises. You cannot sleep when your cortisol is high. When cortisol is high, insulin rises, and high insulin leads to weight gain because insulin is the fat-storing hormone.

Sleep has been provided by nature to do the body's healing work. It takes seven to eight hours for this process to happen. The first three and a half hours are when melatonin is secreted. Then prolactin, which is a pituitary hormone, is released. The National Institutes of Health concludes that six hours of prolactin production in the dark is the minimum necessary to maintain immune function. When prolactin is released, other hormonal functions happen: cortisol goes down, insulin goes down, your thyroid gets a rest as do your adrenals. But if you are imbalanced because your estrogen and progesterone are low or missing due to aging or stress, much less of this healing process can happen.

This is the teeter-totter again: estrogen and progesterone dip, so insulin, cortisol, thyroid, and adrenals rise. One goes down, the others go up.

As a result, insulin stays high, so you gain weight, which can lead to obesity and diabetes—even if you are eating correctly. That is why dieting alone is no longer working for people forty and older. The hormones are no longer in balance and, coupled with your toxic burden, the result is inability to lose weight.

Inability to sleep makes your cortisol rise, making you anxious, and your heart becomes stressed. If your cortisol is high, you can't sleep well. Cortisol is your stress hormone, which is meant to be high only in times of prolonged stress, and even though high cortisol is natural with high stress, it slowly wears away body tissues and good health. High cortisol gives you a "steroid high"; your brain is overactive and you feel pumped up all over. (It's actually adrenaline itself—an entirely separate adrenal hormone from cortisol—that makes the heart pound, not cortisol. And of course adrenaline provides the adrenaline rush. One way to keep these two categorized is to think of adrenaline as the "sprinter's hormone"— rapid onset, only lasts a little while—and of cortisol as the "long distance runner's hormone"—takes longer to get started but can be sustained against stress for much longer before becoming exhausted.) Inability to sleep also diminishes your thyroid, so now you have also diminished fat-burning hormone. Plus the thyroid is responsible for dissolving cholesterol and low thyroid can contribute to autoimmune diseases such as MS and lupus. This cascade, this hormonal crash, throws off your entire system, causing your adrenals to stay revved up and making your heart race, and now sleep becomes impossible.

> You can't sleep because you are in hormonal decline.

Lack of quality sleep leaves you fatigued and depressed and open to disease. It also leads to multiple bodily symptoms, some of which are bloating, hot flashes, and constipation. Your body needs sleep to repair itself and to keep the immune system strong. Yet no one is sleeping and it is happening to younger and younger people. This is a disaster for your health and your weight.

Did you know we were meant to sleep in complete darkness? A recent study put subjects in a completely dark room and then shone little penlights on the backs of their knees. As a result, all the subjects showed raised cortisol levels. Even the smallest amount of light can raise your cortisol levels and just a little extra light could be the thing that is interfering with your ability to sleep. It's important to cover your phone, computer, and TV lights. But most of us keep our lights burning well into the night. We go to sleep surrounded by light from our electronics, phone, and street lamps, and all this light keeps our cortisol from going down.

All of these factors are not conducive to sleeping. They are anti-sleep. This is why millions and millions of Americans are padding around their houses late into the night because they don't sleep in the dark and/or because of hormonal imbalances, and as it is happening, you are getting fatter and fatter.

Think about this. Chronic high cortisol can lead to heart attack or stroke. If you connect the dots, now you understand why the leading killer of women is heart attack . . . but is it?

Hormonal imbalance plays an important role in heart disease in women. Yet daily I hear doctors on the news channels (remember, most doctors only get four hours of instruction in prescribing hormones) speak about the dangers of hormone replacement. These professionals never mention that the hormones they are referring to are artificial hormones, not the natural bioidentical hormones I passionately write about and have personally used for the past twelve blissful years.

So put it all together: We leave the lights on too long, we stay up too late, and we sleep surrounded by lights. We are stressed beyond compare, causing our hormones to decline rapidly. The declining hormones raise our cortisol levels, making sleep impossible. The raised cortisol is accompanied by increased insulin levels, which forces the body to store fat. Then as an added bonus, the thyroid goes low, so there is much less mechanism for fat burning.

And, again, you wonder why you can't lose weight?

EXPERTS WEIGH IN:
A BRIEF INTERVIEW WITH BILL FALOON

The only way to know for sure if your hormones are below optimal levels is to have a blood test or a twenty-four-hour urine test. I have provided numerous resources for doctors on my website, but I have also asked Bill Faloon and his scientific advisory board at *Life Extension* magazine to supply you with an easy and inexpensive way to test your hormone levels. Bill has also given me his thoughts on the connection between balanced hormones and weight loss.

BF: It is true that eating less and avoiding toxic foods addresses many of the underlying causes of weight gain and the accumulation of surplus fat pounds, but it is also partially attributable to the severe alterations that occur in our hormone levels as we age. For instance, a substantial percentage of aging women (and many aging men) have less-than-optimal thyroid levels that predispose them to weight gain. Youthful thyroid hormone levels are needed to maintain healthy metabolic rates, so your body is able to remove fat stores. Those who suffer from a deficiency should be prescribed thyroid hormone replacement. Medications to consider are Armour natural thyroid complex (containing both T4 and T3) or Cytomel (containing T3).

Trying to lose weight in the face of a thyroid deficit can be particularly challenging. However, taking excess amounts of thyroid hormone will not burn away body fat. The objective of testing your blood is to make sure that free T3 levels are in the upper one-third range of normal and that your other thyroid hormone markers are in optimal ranges.

SS: So what should men and women do for optimal balance . . . and weight loss?

BF: A large percentage of men today suffer from abdominal (visceral) obesity, the most dangerous kind of body fat. It is often difficult, if not impossible, for aging men to lose inches off their waistlines if they are deficient in free testosterone, especially in the presence of excess estrogen. Low levels of dehydroepiandrosterone (DHEA) can also contribute to undesirable fat accumulation in men and women.

A comprehensive blood test panel can reveal free testosterone and estrogen levels, and a physician can prescribe a topical testosterone cream and an aromatase inhibitor (to suppress estrogen if necessary) to restore a man's sex hormone profile to a youthful range. The same blood test panel can also detect DHEA blood levels to enable a man to take the proper dose of this over-the-counter dietary supplement.

The benefits of restoring testosterone to youthful ranges extend far beyond losing belly fat. Published scientific studies document a reduction in heart attack risk, alleviation of depression, enhanced sex drive, and a lot more.

A blood test panel for men should also measure prostate-specific antigen (PSA) to help screen for hidden prostate cancer. Those with prostate cancer usually cannot restore their sex hormones until the PSA numbers are lowered.

Some men are able to reduce excess estrogen and simultaneously boost free testosterone by taking nutrient formulas that contain plant extracts to help inhibit the aromatase enzyme (which converts testosterone into estrogen) and decrease levels of sex hormone-binding globulin (which binds free testosterone).

SS: What about women?

BF: A common problem women experience during menopause is an increase in belly fat mass. Estrogen levels plummet during menopause, and some studies correlate this estrogen deficiency with greater abdominal adiposity in women.

While treatment with high dosages of horse-urine-derived estrogens and progestin drugs (Premarin and Provera) may contribute to weight gain, evidence suggests that individually dosed natural (bioidentical) estrogen replacement facilitates a reduction in abdominal fat in women who are estrogen deficient.

Excess levels of testosterone in women can be particularly troublesome, as it can cause abdominal weight gain, which is the opposite of how testosterone works in men. If a woman's blood tests reveal excess levels of free testosterone, there are safe medications that can rapidly bring this hormone into normal ranges.

Restoring hormone balance in aging females requires the intervention of a health care practitioner with specialized expertise in prescribing bioidentical hormone replacement therapy. Men are more fortunate in that most doctors can prescribe the proper dose of testosterone (and aromatase inhibitors if needed).

SS: Anything else you can share?

BF: There is a massive body of scientific data supporting the role that hormones play in regulating body fat storage. To put it simply, hormones tell our cells what to do. In the presence of too much or too little of each of these hormones, aging individuals risk accumulating fat pounds that are difficult to shed.

Fortunately, folks don't have to guess what your hormone status is. You can obtain a male or female hormone blood test panel by going to SuzanneSomers.com and clicking on Life Extension. These tests are offered by Life Extension to Suzanne's readers at a reasonable price. Plus the experts will provide information about the results, and even get you started on a natural hormone balancing program that's right for you.

Here's the solution:

GET HEALTHY, STAY SEXY

- Retrain yourself to go to bed early. Move your bedtime up a little every few days, until you're in bed by 10:00 p.m., or even earlier.

- Try melatonin nightly as a natural sleep aid. Melatonin is a very important hormone we make much less of after around age forty. (It is also a highly potent antioxidant.)

- Take chewable GABA, which can help make sleep deeper and more pleasurable.

- Get a great doc. Find a qualified doctor to prescribe bioidentical hormones and replace what you have lost due to aging and stress.

- Enjoy a Silent Night. Go to SuzanneSomers.com, click on Life-Wave, and order Silent Night sleep patches. They are non-drug patches, and will help you with the retraining of your sleep cycle.

Step 3

USE YOUR GUT
TO LOSE YOUR GUT

I admire Brenda Watson—she is a one-woman crusade for gut health. She is also the author of many books, including some of my favorites: *The H.O.P.E. Formula, The Detox Strategy,* and *The Fiber 35 Diet.* She is one of the foremost authorities in the country on internal cleansing and detoxification. Because of her expertise in digestive health, people flock to her lectures all over the world. Understanding how the gut works is essential to health—and to losing weight—and I asked her to explain the reason why.

SS: So what happens to the gut when a person's diet is genetically modified, full of chemicals, stripped of nutrients, and unvaried? What toll does it take and what can a person expect?

BW: Toxins create gut imbalance, degrade the gut lining, and then enter the circulation, affecting the health of the entire body. Toxins can also enter the body through the lungs and the skin. When the liver can't detoxify them properly, they hide out in unlikely places like the bones, muscles, fat cells, brain tissue, and the liver itself (where they can do serious damage, both in the short term and in the long term). Because many fat-soluble toxins park themselves in fat cells they can mess with signals from these cells that affect our hormones, and that in turn changes our metabolism and how we store (or burn) fat.

SS: It's the point of this book: toxins make you fat. Including the artificial sweeteners in diet sodas that people believe will help them lose weight.

BW: You got that right. What a crock!

SS: It's difficult to make people truly understand that we are facing a chemical and environmental catastrophe regarding our health.

BW: Yes, and more than 60 percent of Americans are also deficient in one or more essential nutrients. The average diet further adds to our toxic load through refined sugars, additives, preservatives, and exposure to pesticides. So eating closer to nature—choosing organically grown foods, high-quality sources of protein, and other nutrients—will offset and support our bodies' natural detoxification system. And weight loss will follow.

SS: That makes sense to me. Let's talk more about gluten intolerance. It is quite the epidemic, and it looks like it is here to stay.

BW: That's for sure. I do want to clarify one thing. Gluten intolerance, or sensitivity, is like a spectrum. Some people are somewhat intolerant and can even eat gluten on a rare occasion. At the other end of the spectrum are people with celiac disease, which is the most severe form. These people must strictly avoid gluten for the rest of their lives or they risk irreversibly damaging their intestinal lining. Celiac disease can be detected by blood tests and intestinal biopsy, while gluten intolerance may be more difficult to pin down.

SS: I understand people of northern European descent are more affected by gluten intolerance. Is that correct?

BW: It used to be that northern Europeans were most affected by gluten, and people of Irish descent were especially affected, but of course now we are seeing gluten intolerance all over the board. And these foods are producing little tiny inflammations that we don't really immediately feel in our gut. It might make its first big appearance with say, chronic fatigue, because this person's gut is now out of balance. But 43 percent of people today are gluten intolerant!

SS: Forty-three percent? That's huge! Is this a result of a lifetime of refined and processed foods, and at a certain point the gut just says, "I give up"?

BW: That and some hereditary markers. Children of alcoholics are at a higher risk. Recently a woman wrote to me and said that she had been on my detox program for a solid year and had some major successes with her lupus, weight gain, migraine headaches, and on and on. She had done the cleansing and the digestive care, but she said something was still missing. She said her face would swell and bloat and she couldn't figure out why. Then she took the test for gluten intolerance and there it was. The puffy face is the giveaway.

It constantly amazes me how many people don't recognize that they are out of balance. Anyone who is overweight is out of balance. And they definitely have a digestion problem, whether they feel it or not.

SS: Do you believe most of this fat is coming from toxins?

BW: Yes, and also a high intake of simple carbohydrates in their diets. You know: cakes, pies, cookies, bread, et cetera.

SS: If I just told people to stop eating cakes, pies, and cookies, it would certainly help, but they still wouldn't get thin because of the toxins in their systems. Will gluten intolerance lead to obesity?

BW: It certainly can. Obesity, simply put, involves being overweight due to excess body fat. About 100 million Americans are overweight. That's one-third of the population. And one-quarter of our children are overweight. It has doubled since the 1980s. Many different proteins and molecules are secreted by fat, so fat now becomes its own organ. The fat tissue is in communication with the rest of your body, especially the endocrine (hormonal) system and the central nervous system. That is why the brain, gut, thyroid, and hormonal connections are vitally important, because you now have a fat organ that is affecting all of these systems.

People who build up fat in their abdominal regions, versus storing it on the hips, are set up to have much greater health consequences. Abdominal fat is connected to the heart, cardiovascular system, liver, and pancreas, which is why we have an epidemic of diabetes. Abdominal fat leads to a condition known as nonalcoholic fatty liver disease (NAFLD), which is associated with metabolic syndrome and can lead to diabetes and heart disease. NAFLD is also associated with gut imbalance. Candida overgrowth increases the production of ethanol (alcohol) in the gut. I can remember years ago I was at a trade show and I talked with Dr. Robert Atkins and he said to me, "The only people I cannot get to lose weight are the people with candida. I have to get rid of that first." Bacterial toxins are also found in the bloodstream of NAFLD patients. All this points to gut imbalance as a contributor to this condition—with the many health implications we've discussed. It's a web of illness, all leading back to the gut.

You can't be healthy if your body can't get nutrients from the foods you eat. Period. So in order to lose weight, your job is to get healthy. And this chapter is about healing an area many don't think of as key in losing weight: the digestive system.

Offending foods play a huge part in weight loss stalls for so many people. If you suspect that foods are making you ill, ask yourself if you are experiencing any of these symptoms:

- Are you constipated?

- Do you have dark circles under your eyes?

- Do you have frequent headaches?

- Do you have joint pain or stiffness?

- Do you feel tired or lethargic?

- Is your hair stringy?

- Does your skin look dull and tired?

- Do you get the flu or colds frequently?

- Do you bloat regularly?

- Do you often have a bad taste in your mouth or bad breath?

- Do you have offensive body odor?

- Does your face sometimes swell?

- Do your feet and ankles ever swell?

- Do you have heartburn or acid reflux?

- Do you have high cholesterol or fatty liver disease?

The more yes responses you have here, the greater the chance you have a food sensitivity or intolerance, and the greater your need to understand the level of your toxic burden and decrease it through natural methods. But first let's take a little tour through our digestive system, as you can't optimize healing if you don't understand how it works.

A LITTLE 411 ON THE GUT

Great health comes from the body's ability to digest nutrients and eliminate waste. The purpose of the digestive system is to be sure you digest your foods completely and eliminate wastes naturally. We are constantly exposed to toxins in our air, food, and water as well as in the workplace and at home, plus we generate toxins in our own bodies. These toxins produce irritation and inflammation, adding to the burden on our digestive system. When the digestive system becomes overwhelmed, it is no longer able to adequately perform detoxification functions. If your gastrointestinal (GI) tract is not working correctly, you won't lose weight easily; it will always be an uphill battle.

In today's world of processed, refined, and chemically sprayed foods, most people are experiencing mild to severe damage to the GI tract. These industrialized and processed foods are hazards to our bodies, as we've already discussed, and are wreaking havoc on our ability to obtain nutrition from what we eat.

Most doctors I have interviewed, as well as reports I have read, all say that disease begins in the GI tract. For our health's sake, we must take the healing of it seriously.

IS YOUR FOOD MAKING YOU SICK?

Food intolerances are a relatively new concept—until very recently, who had ever heard of them? We have always known a few people who were allergic to peanuts or some other food, but today food intolerances are running rampant. And they are causing all kinds of symptoms and reactions: heartburn, migraine headaches, acid reflux, stomachaches, difficulty getting out of bed in the morning, feeling and looking tired even after a good night's sleep, an inability to lose weight, bloating, constipation, relentless water retention. Most people are walking around feeling bad to some degree, but rarely do they make the connection between the symptom and a specific food. As a result of identifying my food sensitivity to eggs and yeast, I was able to easily lose ten pounds simply by giving up the offending foods. And I feel so much better. An allergy or intolerance can be difficult to pinpoint. A compromised immune system is often the result of these intolerances, which compounds the problem for people who already suffer from discomforts caused by certain foods.

ALLERGIES, SENSITIVITIES, AND INTOLERANCES

Food *allergies* are easy to recognize. They involve immediate, strong reactions to foods.

Food *sensitivity* expresses itself in a much subtler way. Food sensitivities are delayed reactions to foods; they can occur anywhere from a few hours to a few days after exposure. They can become health problems, with a full-blown reaction every time you eat the offending food, if the toxic load is too heavy.

An allergic response is generally limited to the air passages, skin, and digestive tract. For example, when someone eats strawberries and develops hives, or is exposed to pollen and starts sneezing, this is a classic allergic response, the type for which allergists test with skin pricks. This type of reaction is an immunoglobulin E (IgE) antibody-mediated reaction to antigens in the food.

Food sensitivity, in contrast to an acute allergic response, is caused by immunoglobulin G (IgG) and may affect any organ or tissue of the body, resulting in a wide array of physical and emotional symptoms. Such reactions can be delayed by as much as three days, so they are frequently not recognized as food sensitivities.

It is common for reactive foods to be consumed
frequently to the point of addiction. Case in point:
alcoholics. By habitually consuming foods (here,
alcohol) that the body doesn't want, the person
unconsciously avoids withdrawal symptoms.

Unfortunately, eating foods your body rejects will perpetuate digestive disorders. When the food-sensitive person eats the offending foods on a daily basis, the small intestine responds by producing an antibody response. With the passing of time this response irritates the digestive lining by producing inflammation. The response is analogous to wearing wool every day; the skin would eventually react by becoming inflamed. The same holds true for the lining of the gut.

Dr. Nicholas Gonzalez, a dear friend whom I featured in my book *Knockout,* said recently, "There is an epidemic of gluten and wheat sensitivity in modern times. This is becoming an increasing problem, and for a very simple reason. Forty years ago, farmers, organic or otherwise, had access to some one hundred different varieties of wheat, each with its own particular value and each with a particular soil proclivity, et cetera. Most of these were very easy to digest. However, with the advent of high-tech farming and very selective breeding, farmers now have access to generally only five strains, all of which are very hardy and all of which are more difficult for humans to digest. This applies to organic as well as nonorganic farms. This has been a particular problem in the past ten years. As a result, even people with no history of gluten or wheat sensitivity are showing symptoms. What's changed isn't their metabolism but the reliance on a limited number of tough-to-digest strains of wheat—even in the organic marketplace. It's a vastly underappreciated problem."

FROM A SWEET TOOTH TO FULL-BLOWN ALLERGIES: MY GRANDDAUGHTER'S STORY

She's an incredible child, Bruce and Caroline's oldest daughter, Camelia. I was in the delivery room when she was born. In fact, as the doctor was performing the C-section, Camelia was only halfway out of the womb, and I held her little hand—creating a connection between the three generations that cannot be shaken.

A healthy and energetic child, Camelia has always been on the go. Very active, bright, funny—and man, does she love her sugar. I used to joke that she inherited my sweet tooth. She started having some health problems in fourth grade—stomachaches that could not be traced to a particular food or activity or to stress. They were located in the upper abdomen; sometimes after she ate, sometimes on an empty stomach, sometimes after exercise, sometimes in bed. On occasion she would complain of pains in her chest, like she was having a heart attack. We were obviously concerned. The pediatrician did tests; her digestive tract was clean. He tried taking her off dairy; no results. Over time the episodes tapered off somewhat, but when they came she just learned to live with them.

One day in sixth grade she called home to say half of her face was numb, including her tongue; she had numbness in her right hand, and she was speaking in jumbled phrases and transposing her letters as she wrote. Caroline immediately called a neurologist, who told her that when he hears about those symptoms in adults he thinks stroke, but in kids he thinks migraine. Caroline rushed to pick her up. By the time she got there, Camelia had an intense pain behind her eye, and fell fast asleep on the way to the neurologist's office. This was a classic migraine headache—her first one, at only age eleven. After getting some background information, the doctor was immediately able to connect the dots regarding her stomachaches back in fourth grade—they were "abdominal migraines." And the pains shooting up her chest were part of the nerve path.

Finally we had a piece to the puzzle. She had a diagnosis, but what was causing the migraines? Hormone fluctuations? She was getting close to that age. After she had several debilitating episodes, I asked Dr. Jonathan Wright for his thoughts, and he immediately suspected allergies, specifically gluten and dairy. He had seen the connection of adolescent migraines with gluten and dairy allergies many times before. He suggested Caroline and Bruce give Camelia magnesium oil to prevent the migraines, explaining that this deficiency is common among migraine sufferers. They ordered the magnesium oil and rubbed a small amount on her forearm every day, and the migraines seemed to taper off.

The following year, Caroline called me, again concerned about Camelia. She was getting bloated, particularly in the face and stomach. This is a kid who dances three hours a day, so where was this swelling coming from? Something was off. The clincher was one night when Camelia had a severe allergic reaction to a cat—the first time in her life. Her whole face blew up. Now it seemed an allergy test was a necessity.

Dr. Wright ordered a blood and stool test (which checks another type of antibody called IgA), explaining that many allergies to gluten are missed in blood tests (which check the IgG antibody) alone. He also ordered a mineral test on her hair and a candida test. Bingo—when the results came back, Camelia was off-the-charts allergic to gluten, dairy, eggs, several kinds of nuts, soy, beef, pineapple, peaches, and many more things she regularly ate. Dr. Wright explained that with gluten sensitivity, the body does not absorb nutrition, so even though you are eating, you are not getting the amino acids, minerals, and many other nutrients the body needs for fuel. That's why Camelia had such a huge craving for sugar! When people have gluten allergy, eating that sugar means survival. And they keep eating it to fuel their bodies.

He explained that Camelia was so full of antibodies to various allergens that her body was basically at war all the time fighting them. The cumulative effect had caused something called leaky gut syndrome. This means that some of the allergic substances were leaking into the bloodstream, where the second line of defense—white blood cells—then started making those IgG antibodies. He described them as being like criminals who had escaped from jail and were marauding in the streets. All that warfare between allergens and antibodies in the system contribute to inflammation and other disruption, which explained the bloating and weight gain. How about the cat reaction? She only reacted to the cat because her total allergen load (from the food allergies) was so high that when a respiratory allergen came along, like the cat, it was a tipping point. Without the food allergies, she never would have reacted to that cat. Her candida test turned out to be negative—that was good. But in her intestine he did find abnormal types and amounts of bacteria, which also cause inflammation. Her mineral tests showed she was low in a number of essential minerals, indicating she had had this gluten sensitivity for a long time and it was wreaking havoc on her system. Had we not caught this problem, Camelia's bones would likely have deteriorated to full-blown osteoporosis by the time she was only in her forties! And if the gluten allergy continued to go unchecked, she could have destroyed her digestive system and ended up with ulcerative colitis (another often gluten-related disease) by eighteen.

Here is the program Dr. Wright suggested for her: eliminate all the foods on the upper scale of the allergy test, eat the foods in the midrange no more than once every four days, and enjoy the foods in the low range at will. This was a huge adjustment for Camelia, but she is lucky to have a mother who prepares fresh protein and vegetables anyway. It meant getting rid of the junk she liked to eat for treats, and avoiding all that stuff served at school and parties. Not easy for a fourteen-year-old kid, but Camelia wanted her health and her body back. In addition, she takes powdered glutamine plus probiotics every morning and evening to help repair the intestinal damage caused by the gluten allergy, and a customized blend of amino acids to rebuild her muscles and other protein-containing tissues. For about eight weeks he also prescribed goldenseal to reduce the abnormal bacteria in her intestine (this was the natural alternative to giving her an antibiotic). She saw an almost immediate decrease in bloating once she started this. And to round out her overall health, she took a multivitamin, vitamin D (5,000 IU), vitamin K, calcium, and Lugol's iodine for breast cancer prevention (7 drops once a week).

I am so proud of how cooperative Camelia has been. It's no easy task. In time, Dr. Wright says, she can become desensitized to most of the allergy

foods—with the exception of gluten. The gluten allergy is a genetic predisposition and she will never be able to eat gluten without adverse effects to
her health. For most of his life, my son, Bruce, has had horrible respiratory
allergies; Dr. Wright suspects his allergies are underlied by a gluten sensitivity and that he passed this down to Camelia. He also suggested that
my younger granddaughter, Violet, get tested. Guess what? She's allergic
to gluten, dairy, and eggs. Fortunately, hers was caught before major damage to her system. In the meantime, Camelia is slowly seeing and feeling
the results and has adapted to this new lifestyle. Thank you, Dr. Wright.
From the first time I told him she had a migraine, he suspected gluten and
dairy! It is a privilege to work with such excellent doctors and to share
these findings with my readers.

Perhaps the gut discomfort you have been experiencing all your life
has been a food intolerance, sensitivity, or allergy that started as a child.
This is why I have included Camelia's story. Had this gone unchecked,
she could have ended up with Crohn's disease due to gluten intolerance. Maybe this has been your impediment to losing weight your entire
life. If her symptoms resonate with you, then it will serve you well to be
tested for sensitivities or intolerances.

Both sensitivities and allergies can develop in response to anything in
the environment, not just food. The offending substance might be corn,
petrochemicals, or any of the numerous toxins that now contaminate the
planet. The response to these antigens can affect any organ of the body,
but the gut will always be involved. Poor digestion and food sensitivities
are tied together. The more food allergies or sensitivities a person has, the
more the body reacts and triggers the immune system to activate inflammation throughout the body (especially in the GI tract).

Also, the improper digestion of food can lead to an allergy-like response.
When undigested food particles enter the circulation through the walls of
the intestine, the body responds as if they were foreign invaders, forming
what are known as immune complexes. Brenda Watson says: "Immune
complexes are formed when an antibody binds to a water soluble anti-

gen. Clusters of these antibody antigens are immune complexes. They are cleared from the body via the macrophages in the spleen or the Kupffer cells of the liver. If this does not happen, they circulate in the blood and are deposited in the organs or joints, and they can cause autoimmune disease. For example, in people who are gluten sensitive, the gluten becomes an antigen and can create these immune complexes by the binding of the antibody formed in reaction to gluten. If the liver or spleen is not strong enough to clear these complexes, then inflammation occurs. This can also happen with other toxins."

THE CONNECTION TO WEIGHT LOSS

Food allergies and food sensitivities, along with toxic exposure, are yet another piece of the puzzle of why you can't lose weight. You eat the offending food, it creates a toxic reaction, the toxicity drains your energy, you crave fattening and sugary foods to get some energy as an unconscious means of survival, and the offending food weakens your immune system, leaving you susceptible to various diseases. When you feel weakened, what quicker way to get energy than with bad carbs, sugar, or processed foods with chemicals? At this point, the body has no choice but to store the toxins in fat—everything that enters through your mouth or the skin must be used, eliminated, or stored, and since toxins can't be used and your weakened lymphatic system means they cannot be easily eliminated, the body has little choice but to store them in fat. The more toxins you take in, the more fat you need for storage. Another vicious cycle. Now do you see that the more toxic the body becomes, the fatter you get . . . and the sicker?

According to Dr. James Breneman's *Basics of Food Allergy*, published in 1978 when Dr. Breneman was chair of the Food Allergy Committee of the American College of Allergists—the number one professional organization for allergists in the United States—food allergy and sensitivity can cause arthritis, bursitis, low-back pain, hives, eczema, itching, asthma, fainting, flushing, dizzy spells, bedwetting, recurrent bladder infection, canker sores, low blood sugar, diarrhea, attacks of gallbladder pain, aggravations of diabetes, indigestion, acid reflux and heartburn, constipation, abdominal bloating, crankiness, other personality changes, migraine headache, fatigue, learning disability, puffiness in the hands, feet, and face, and rapid water retention of up to 4 percent of body weight.

One easy way to determine if you're food allergic or sensitive is to weigh yourself every day. If you gain two pounds or more overnight, it's obviously water weight, fluid retention caused by food allergy or sensitivity. Fat doesn't store that rapidly! Caution: Not everyone sensitive or allergic to food gains water weight; this self-test only finds food allergy or sensitivity for some of us.

I remember when one of my dear friends started having trouble with swelling feet and ankles. They would blow up so badly she could hardly walk. Once she took off her shoes, getting them back on was virtually impossible. Her stomach would also bloat. She had always been lean and lithe, even though she ate sugar night and day and drank Coke constantly. She was thin, so it never seemed to be a problem taking in so much sugar, like it is for the rest of us. But once this discomfort and swelling began (which I now realize was inflammation running amok) it never went away. It continued for years, and she gained a little more weight each year. I never thought much about it at the time, but now I realize that those were the first warning signs of an immune system that was breaking down from toxicity and no one understood the trigger.

Was an accumulated toxic burden in her body finally rearing its ugly head? Was it the enormous amounts of sugar she consumed? Was it hormonal imbalance? Or was it all of the above? Were these the early warning signs indicating issues that for her would one day end up as lung cancer and emphysema? Was it just bad luck, or was it toxicity and allergies?

Could it have been sensitivity to corn, sugar, dairy, or gluten? Swollen feet and ankles are indicators. A simple test early on would have identified the offending foods, and she might have been able to reverse the problems . . . if only we had known.

My Husband Alan's Story

From my earliest memories, I had serious stomach problems. In grade school, I would go to the nurse's office with a bloated and aching stomach, and the diagnosis was always the same: spasmodic stomach, whatever that means. It never stopped, but it now had a name. All my life, until just a few years ago, I carried that awful burden. Even though I ate organic food, replaced my hormones, loaded up with supplements, and had a great marriage and family, my stomach bloated every afternoon around three o'clock, and sometimes I had to go to sleep from exhaustion. Why was I so exhausted? I slept eight to nine hours nightly. Then one of my many tests came back, and there it was; a serious gluten intolerance, with celiac disease just around the corner. I stopped all gluten instantly, and I have not bloated since then. And I am no longer exhausted in the middle of the afternoon, either. I lost 3 inches off my waist and my love handles all but disappeared. The biggest surprise was that my food intake dropped in half; I had been eating double the amount of food because the gluten problem did not permit proper absorption of nutrients. Once I stopped all gluten, I was a happy fellow. Almost half the population is gluten intolerant, but they don't know it. They do what I did for most of my life: simply accept the fact that every day brings discomfort. I suggest everyone over forty get tested. It'll change lives.

SO WHAT CAN YOU DO?

The good news is that a simple blood test is available to check for food allergies, sensitivities, and intolerances. It will all be done in the same test. Go to SuzanneSomers.com and click on Life Extension. They offer this test at a reasonable price and will interpret the results for you.

My husband took this blood test and it changed his life. He never realized how bad he felt after eating certain foods until after he stopped eating

What You Need to Know About Gluten

Gluten is a special type of protein found in rye, wheat, barley, spelt, triticale, and kamut. Therefore it is found in most types of cereal and in many types of bread. Gluten is also found in oats, but there is debate among physicians about whether oat gluten causes the same problems as gluten from other grains. Not all foods from the grain family, however, contain gluten. Wild rice, corn, buckwheat, millet, quinoa, teff, soybeans, and sunflower seeds don't have it. A gluten sensitivity is a condition in which an individual experiences an adverse reaction to the consumption of any substance containing gluten proteins. A gluten sensitivity can overlap many of the same symptoms as celiac disease. In cases of celiac disease, the reaction to gluten is obvious, sometimes with constipation, sometimes with multiple stools daily, diarrhea, gas, bloating, and cramps. Celiac disease is sometimes severe. What distinguishes gluten sensitivity from celiac disease is that someone with this type of food sensitivity is often able to consume small and infrequent amounts of gluten-containing products without exhibiting a severe reaction. By contrast, an individual suffering with celiac would have to avoid gluten in any form or run the risk of serious repercussions each and every time even a tiny amount of gluten is consumed.

If you are suffering from either gluten intolerance or celiac disease, you might wonder, what can you eat? A lot.

Gluten-free grains, including rice, wild rice, corn, buckwheat, millet, quinoa, teff, and sometimes oats (also, oats can be contaminated by wheat products during processing, so make sure to look for "gluten-free" products to avoid cross-contamination); unlimited amounts of vegetables; all fruits; all beans; all nuts; all poultry (chicken, turkey, duck, etc.), fish, and seafood. As far as dairy goes, most everyone can tolerate butter, but a test for milk allergy and sensitivity and a separate test for lactose intolerance (the former usually involves milk proteins, the latter milk sugar) is advised to be sure you can tolerate other cow products. Cheeses and yogurt made from sheep's or goat's milk, however, are allowed. As for oils, flaxseed, hemp, avocado, extra virgin olive, and perilla are all good choices. Eggs are another great choice, unless an intolerance to them appears in your blood work. Most gluten intolerants can handle oat milk, almond milk, or rice milk. Extremely sensitive gluten intolerants may have a much wider range of food restrictions, which will be revealed in your test results.

gluten. Years of bloating and discomfort, fatigue, the need for frequent naps, unexplained weight gain, and a loss of vitality and energy—all was rectified once he gave up the offending foods.

For people with sensitivities (depending on the degree) the smallest bit of the offending food can cause a reaction like, say, a mini spoonful of poison. Who would feel well taking any amount of poison?

But how can we know if we are sensitive to or intolerant to any foods? The abovementioned blood test can identify many of the offenders. When my granddaughter took the allergy test we were shocked at the breadth of her sensitivities: everything from gluten and dairy to soy, brown rice, pinto beans, and countless other foods. Dr. Jonathan Wright was able to interpret her tests for her and asked that she give up all the offending foods until her body calmed down and was able to detoxify. Gluten was the only exception: she was so sensitive to it that he told her most likely she could never have gluten foods again.

According to Brenda Watson, there are certain foods you have to be careful of if you're gluten intolerant, as these foods may be hidden sources of gluten:

- Modified food starch

- Thickening agents

- Caramel coloring

- MSG

- Malted milk

- Flavored and instant coffees

- Soy sauce

- Emulsifiers

- Stabilizers

- Hydrolyzed vegetable proteins

- Packaged rice mixes

- Creamed vegetables

- Nondairy creamers

- Prepared meats (sandwich meats, hot dogs)

- Premade salad dressings

- Vodka, whiskey, beer, gin, wine, malt liquor

- Ovaltine

- Ice cream

- Bouillon cubes

- Chocolate

- Catsup

- Pie fillings

- Baking powders

- Chewing gum

- Dry seasoning mixes

- Gravy mixes

- Processed cheeses

- Packaged dips

- Vanilla and flavorings made with alcohol

- Most condiments

CELLULITE OR FOOD ALLERGY?

Hate your cellulite? Think cellulite is a fait accompli that accompanies aging? Well, not necessarily so. Cellulite is most often caused by allergic reactions and an immune response to food proteins. A delayed allergic reaction to offending foods occurs within blood vessels, causing inflammation in the vessel walls, which subsequently can trigger clotting mechanisms. This increased inflammation in the arteries and capillaries contributes to poor circulation, which is a known cause of cellulite, and reduced lymphatic drainage. Avoiding food intolerances will diminish the appearance of cellulite and stop its formation for good . . . another great reason to eliminate toxins and toxic foods from your system!

WHAT ABOUT MILK?

Milk allergy is allergy or sensitivity to milk proteins, inclucing casein, lactoglobulin, lactalbumin, and many others. IgG and other antibodies are involved in milk allergy and can be detected by the blood test available through Life Extension (see Resources).

Not everyone who has lactose sensitivity also has a milk protein allergy, and not everyone with milk protein allergy has lactose sensitivity. Since most hard cheeses have their milk sugar fermented away, people who have lactose intolerance can sometimes eat cheeses without problems, while people with milk allergy often can't.

LISTEN TO YOUR BODY

Many people are suffering from symptoms of fibromyalgia, lupus, rheumatoid arthritis, or other diseases and autoimmune responses, never realizing their connection to possible allergies or our toxic burden, and that detoxification would most likely alleviate many of these symptoms and often prevent them in the first place.

> The body talks!
> It is we who don't listen to its language.

Uncovering food sensitivities is a powerful process. Once you have determined the effects of particular foods on your health, you have to decide if it's worth it or not to eat them. There are some people, like my granddaughter, who find that even a crumb will affect them; others, like my husband, can occasionally tolerate a little gluten, but to indulge too often is asking for trouble. It's not just the discomfort food sensitivities create in the body but what these offender foods can bring long-term in the form of serious disease. Some doctors tell me that, unfortunately, cancer is one of them. Weight gain is another. Many cutting-edge doctors, as well as myself, believe that toxins and food sensitivities are likely at the base of most unexplained weight gain.

LEAKY GUT SYNDROME

The health of the gastrointestinal tract is dependent on healthy food choices. Consuming and breathing chemicals creates an imbalance of bacteria, insufficient enzymes, low hydrochloric acid levels, and out-of-control inflammation. Any one of these factors may result in an irritation of the digestive wall. When that happens tiny holes may form, allowing partially digested material, toxins, or bacteria to pass through. This is called *leaky gut syndrome*.

Leaky gut is serious and causes symptoms of digestive upset, gas, bloating, pain, and weakened immunity. According to Dr. Jonathan Wright, several supplements can help repair a damaged digestive tract wall. These include:

- Aloe vera

- Butyrate (particularly for the colon)

- Calendula

- Chamomile

- Deglycyrrhizinated licorice (DGL)

- Glutamine

- Marshmallow (the supplement, not the fluffy kind in the plastic bag)

- Plantain

- Vitamin A (never take more than 10,000 IU if there's any chance you might become pregnant)

- Zinc

With the exception of butyrate, glutamine, vitamin A, and zinc, these supplements are known as demulcents because they help coat and heal the digestive tract, and most of us can use help to repair our gut wall.

Leaky gut is exacerbated by severe stress. I know firsthand. A decade ago when my mother passed I never allowed myself to properly grieve and deal with my emotional pain. Right after her funeral I jumped back into full work mode. It was avoidance for sure, thinking I could bury myself in my projects and not feel this terrible loss, but the body and the cells have an intelligence much greater than that of the conscious mind. Eventually my body came to a screeching halt by developing symptoms of unbelievable fatigue and depression, forcing me to slow down and finally grieve. The exhaustion became so overwhelming I could not walk the short way upstairs to my bedroom without stopping halfway to rest. I would fall asleep if I happened to sit down for even a few minutes—once I even fell asleep on the air while on the Home Shopping Network. It felt like my body was coming to an end, as though I was completely out of gas. Finally it became alarming, so I went to my doctor; he diagnosed leaky gut. He took me off all sugar and alcohol, put me on an IV detox regimen of glutathione and vitamin C, created a supplement regimen, and strongly advised for my health's sake that I take it seriously, which I did. It took almost a year to repair the damage.

> There are no shortcuts to true health.

It wasn't about pills or pharmaceuticals. Healing required a new focus on healthy eating, getting eight hours of sleep each night, and avoiding sugar and other offending foods.

Part of detoxing my body involved going for regular colonics. It was all part of cleaning out the toxic burden I now realized I carried within, and one day during the process the floodgates opened. I lay on that table and cried like a baby. I guess it's not so strange that it would happen during a detoxification, but finally I allowed the grief to manifest. From that time on, along with the health regimen I had adopted, I got well . . . and I got thin. This experience was invaluable to me. I began listening to my body and recognizing that even the smallest symptoms are the body's language . . . the warning signs.

FIBER AND PROBIOTICS: TWO KEY WEAPONS IN HEALING AND WEIGHT LOSS

Fiber

We hear a lot about the benefits of fiber and probiotics, but there is still confusion as to why they are relevant and important to our health . . . and to our ability to control our weight.

Constipation plagues most American adults at some time or another. Eating dietary fiber is one way to get and stay regular. The muscles of the colon need to be exercised in order to stay fit. Dietary fiber in the digestive tract creates bulk to keep these muscles working and make them strong and healthy. Years of consuming too little fiber causes the muscles of the colon to become weak and atrophied, with chronic constipation as a result; this is compounded by the fact that many people do not drink enough water. Eight glasses of water a day might seem overwhelming, but it is one of the best ways to stay regular, lose weight, and detoxify. Start by making it a point to drink a glass of water every hour over eight of the hours of the day. You won't believe the results. Your skin will look better, your bowels will move easily and regularly, and you will wash out toxins and keep your colon hydrated.

According to Michael Murray, ND, the average daily fiber consumption in the United States is approximately 20 grams per person. Such a low fiber intake results in a digestive transit time of forty-eight hours or more, and this slow exit can result in the absorption of toxins from putrefied fecal material that has not been eliminated. (I know—yuck!)

The absorption of toxins from within the body's digestive system is a form of self-poisoning that can lead to serious disease and, again, weight gain. The weight comes from the accumulated toxins that result from not eliminating properly, and as we know by now toxins have nowhere to be stored but—you guessed it—fat. The more you are constipated, the more toxic you become. But fiber is a non-nutritive food component that provides bulk and helps move food residue through the intestines, reducing the absorbtion of toxins. Fiber is found naturally in whole grains, fruits, and vegetables. When whole grains are refined (think white flour, white rice), out go the benefits of the fiber that would have been part of that food.

Health expert Brenda Watson says we should get at least 35 grams of fiber daily. Aim for that from your food, and if you can't eat that much fiber comfortably, see the Resources section for a good source of additive fiber.

It is important to note that fiber will not correct everyone's constipation problems. Some people suffer from insufficient peristalsis, which means muscles in their colon do not sufficiently contract to achieve complete elimination. Drinking a buffered vitamin C powder (using magnesium or potassium as the buffering agent) on an empty stomach several days a week can naturally stimulate peristalsis to evacuate fecal accumulation.

Probiotics: How the Right Bacteria Can Help

The word *probiotic* literally means "for life." What are probiotics, though? They are good bacteria (yes, bacteria) that aid us in health and healing. Why should you care? Probiotic supplements help keep a healthy balance of beneficial bacteria in your digestive tract, which is home to more than five hundred different species of bacteria. Good bacteria are critical in your body's ability to deflect incoming toxins and aid the body's elimination of them. This is what we are looking for. We are trying to lose weight, and to do so, we need to find as many ways as we can to eliminate toxins. It all adds up. Eliminate toxins here and there and pretty soon you are reducing your toxic burden. You will see it on your body, thinner and healthier.

According to the *American Journal of Clinical Nutrition*, good bacteria crowd out disease-producing bacteria, allow us to better absorb our vitamins (especially B vitamins and vitamin K), help us to produce natural antibodies that kill pathogenic (disease-producing) bacteria, help the body make short-chain fatty acids to promote good colon function, increase fecal bulking, promote mineral absorption, and may help prevent colon cancer. In short, probiotics strengthen your immune system, help maintain a healthy colon, help the body digest food, and create an unfriendly environment for harmful bacteria and yeast. In essence, just as their name suggests, probiotics are life-promoting.

We get much of the good bacteria we need daily from our diet, but as we age, the amount of our good bacteria naturally decreases. Fermented dairy and vegetable foods such as yogurt, kefir, and sauerkraut are all high in good bacteria (but only if not heated to high temperature, which tends to destroy the good bacteria). Eating those foods is very beneficial, especially when coupled with a high-fiber diet, because good bacteria love to eat soluble fiber. Why is that a good thing?

Soluble fiber absorbs toxins as it passes through the GI tract and slows down the absorption of nutrients. This keeps blood sugar levels down, which in turn keeps your appetite in check and takes away sugar cravings. Either way, you get the skinny.

Insoluble fiber moves bulk through the intestines and controls and balances the pH (acidity) in the intestines. When good bacteria multiply they crowd out the bad bacteria and create balance. If you are not getting enough good bacteria from your diet, you can supplement with a high-potency supplement. I take one capsule a day of bifidobacteria with the right amount of lactobacilli. (These can be purchased at a health food store or at RenewLife.com.)

ENZYME BALANCE

The next component to a healthy GI tract is enzyme balance.

In my last book, *Knockout,* Dr. Nicholas Gonzalez talked about the critical need for enzyme replacement for his cancer patients. Enzymes are protein-based substances that are essential to every function in the human body: eating, digesting, absorbing, seeing, hearing, smelling, breathing, kidney function, liver function, reproduction, elimination, and more. Plus, enzymes are powerful little workers in removing toxins from your body.

Dr. Gonzalez feels that if a body requires healing, then restoring enzyme balance is crucial. For health's sake, enzymes are crucial for removing toxins, and when you detoxify with enzymes you will have another weapon in your Sexy Forever arsenal to make you healthy and thin.

The best way to get enzymes is to eat fresh fruits and vegetables daily. But the enzymatic content of fresh foods diminishes with long-term storage, as well as from pesticides and toxins in the water and soil. Also, an aging body has decreased enzyme activity, so supplementation is something to consider. Brenda Watson says, "Normally enzymes are present in raw foods to assist in digestion, but many foods get depleted of their natural enzymes through cooking and processing. Without the essential enzymes needed for proper digestion, the body can't break down those foods to absorb their nutrients. As a result, undigested food in the digestive tract can ferment, causing gas, bloating, and other digestive difficulties. Supplementing with digestive enzymes will decrease the need for all of the pancreatic enzyme secretions to be active in the digestive tract. This will allow some of the pancreatic enzymes to be absorbed into the blood, where they can work on that portion of food that enters the blood and lymphatic system undigested, helping to break it down."

Remember, everything suggested in this book is to help you unload your toxic burden, so that you can gain control over your health. To be healthy and thin you must understand all the opportunities you have to detoxify your life. While it's impossible to detox every aspect of your life, having this information allows you to chip away where you can. If you do this, your weight will find its perfect balance for your ideal body composition.

A WORD ON HYDROCHLORIC ACID

I discussed the importance of hydrochloric acid (HCL) in my book *Breakthrough*, but it bears repeating. HCL is produced by parietal cells (tiny pumps) in the lining of the stomach, and this acid is needed to ensure the proper functioning of the stomach. HCL has at least two primary functions: it provides the acidic environment necessary for the enzyme pepsin to break down proteins, and it helps prevent infection by destroying most parasites and bacteria.

Most people with heartburn produce too little hydrochloric acid, yet the usual remedy is to take an antacid, which removes acid—exactly the opposite of what your stomach wants! So throw away those little cherry-flavored over-the-counter antacids or prescription acid blockers. They are doing you harm. Your stomach actually needs hydrochloric acid to help nourish your body! Without enough HCL, you may not be able to sufficiently break down proteins. This can lead to bloating, gas, and, you guessed it, more heartburn. Low HCL production can also result in problems with bacterial infections or parasites.

Your body once made sufficient and in some cases abundant HCL. Aging can knock out most of the HCL in your digestive system. This decline begins around age forty, and from then on, many people suffer the effects of low stomach acid. Because of powerful advertising, they feel that the remedy is to pop down those cherry-flavored antacids like candy, but that only covers up symptoms and doesn't fix the basic problem. Once your body is no longer making sufficient HCL the only way to restore it is through supplementation. Supplemental HCL is available in tablet form. Supplementation will keep you feeling good. And best of all it will be one of the crucial steps in eliminating bloating. Yay! As Dr. Wright and Dr. Lenard say in their book *Why Stomach Acid Is Good for You,* "We should always try to copy nature!"

Low stomach acid leads to weight gain because your food is not digesting properly, which creates toxins that then get stored (you guessed it again) in the fat. More toxins, more fat. Without HCL you will become bloated, constipated, and unable to extract nutrients from your food. If you go to your regular doctor he may prescribe Nexium or Prilosec for your heartburn and acid reflux, which again is a bandage and will never heal you. In addition, you are also adding to your toxic burden. Instead, natural hydrochloric acid is available in tablet form at your local health food store and will replace the missing component, allowing you to properly digest your food, while eliminating acid reflux. Chronic, persistent acid reflux—even if the amount of acid made by the stomach is actually too low—can lead to esophageal cancer, so take it seriously.

Hydrochloric acid is crucial for my personal gut health, so I take three capsules with every meal. Radiation (which I had for my cancer) knocked out my body's ability to manufacture HCL *for life*. The type of HCL I take is called betaine HCL.

The properly functioning stomach secretes at least five important substances: mucus, hydrochloric acid, a digestive enzyme called pepsin, an acid-regulating hormone called gastrin, and gastric lipase, which assists in the digestion of fat. Here's why you need to understand this mechanism. Mucus coats the cells lining the stomach to protect them from the HCL. This mucus can be damaged by dehydration, overconsumption of food or aspirin, or by the bacterium *Helicobacter pylori* (*H. pylori*).

Many people are walking around with *H. pylori* without realizing it, yet the symptoms of bloating and discomfort persist, regardless of how well they eat. Unchecked, *H. pylori* can lead to damage of the mucosal lining, and this damage can often lead to gastritis, which is an irritation of the stomach lining. It can even lead to a stomach ulcer. *H. pylori* is a bad bacterium that produces substances that are harmful to the body. It irritates the lining of the intestines (causing gas) and can be absorbed into the bloodstream (causing disease). It cannot be prevented from entering the body, but if the number of good bacteria stays high, then the *H. pylori* will be kept to a minimum. Another example of bad bacteria is *salmonella*. Both *H. pylori* and salmonella can lead to serious disease, a kind of poisoning of the body. It's important to rule out both of them and other bad bacteria through proper testing. In with the good bacteria, out with the bad. Your body and health will thank you for it.

A Good NAG

Much of the mucus lining of the gut contains the amino sugar N-acetyl-glucosamine (NAG). L-glutamine exists in virtually all cells, and it is one of the most prevalent amino acids in the body. Humans must have L-glutamine in order to produce NAG and have a healthy mucosal lining. If you eat at restaurants frequently and order chicken a lot, you are likely to have been exposed to *H. pylori*. Unfortunately, *H. pylori* have the unique capability of navigating their way right through mucous, gastric or otherwise. I feel I have a better shot at avoiding bacteria or *H. pylori* when I buy organic chicken for home preparation. I always eat organic food at home (on the road it's not so easy to avoid the hazards of poor-quality food). A good qualified doctor will understand how to treat this condition. (Go to SuzanneSomers.com for listings.) If you do have *H. pylori,* taking supplements of NAG (N-acetyl-glucosamine) is an important remedy.

GETTING THIN FOR LIFE

We already discussed how important good nutrition is. If your body is not able to extract nutrients via your GI tract, you will get increasingly unhealthy regardless of how well you eat. If you are nutritionally void because of poor food choices, coupled with a diet that is heavy in chemicals, you will gradually feel worse. Plus you'll get fatter and fatter, and eventually you will get sick. Are you getting the connection? More toxins require more fat for storage. I will say this over and over: it's the toxic buildup that is keeping you fat.

GET HEALTHY, STAY SEXY

In summary, if you have problems with your digestive health, you must first heal your gut in order to lose weight and get healthy:

- Take a blood test for food sensitivities and food allergies. Also ask for a celiac disease screening panel that contains deamidated gliadin IgA, tissue transglutaminase IgA, and serum IgA.

  You can obtain a convenient walk-in test for food intolerances/allergies by logging on to SuzanneSomers.com and clicking on Life Extension.

- Eliminate toxic chemicals from your life as best you can.

- Take supplements to heal the GI tract: glutamine, deglycyrrhinated licorice (DGL), aloe vera, plantain, marshmallow, gamma-lipoic acid.

- For leaky gut, see a qualified doctor for a list of supplements, and ask about IV glutathione and vitamin C.

- Consider wearing LifeWave glutathione patches to detoxify.

- Balance your enzymes.

- If needed, replace missing hydrochloric acid with each meal.

- Take N-acetyl-glucosamine (NAG) if you have *H. pylori* bacteria.

- Consume at least 35 grams of fiber daily to alleviate constipation and keep the GI tract healthy.

- Take probiotics. Look for a capsule that has 80 billion bifidobacteria and lactobacilli.

- Supplement daily with cod liver oil or good-quality omega-3 oil, and always use good-quality oils in your cooking.

These changes will have a dramatic effect on your health, and the stubborn weight that just won't seem to go away will begin to melt off, provided you are following the Sexy Forever plan. Real food, real weight loss, and real health. What more could you want?

Following all of these steps is important. Just watching what you eat is, sad to say, no longer enough. As I have said and will say over and over, the planet has changed, and either you accept it and make adjustments or you go the way of others you see around you and become overweight and sick. Make the decision to win this war of toxins versus our bodies. It *is* possible.

Step 4

ALL THE RIGHT MOVES

From middle age on there is nothing more vital to your health and weight control than to build lean muscle mass, and the only way that happens is with weight training and exercise. Exercise brings remarkable benefits. And although it is not essential for weight loss, the increased calorie burn from muscle makes you lose weight faster than you would otherwise.

The reason most people tend to gain a few pounds each year after age thirty is that unless we take specific steps to stop lean muscle mass from declining, it will slide, leaving you with less calorie-burning muscle and more fat. Then you are in a vicious cycle: less lean muscle causes you to burn fewer calories, and if you continue eating badly, you will continue to gain weight. Unless you exercise to maintain or increase your lean muscle, you will gain weight every year.

Exercise builds more than muscle; it builds health. Sitting around and watching TV instead of getting up and getting some exercise sets up a chain reaction for deterioration and poor health. A sedentary lifestyle reduces your ability to take in and use oxygen. If you take in less oxygen, you get less oxygen in your blood. Less oxygen in your blood means less oxygen in the cells, which means less energy and vitality in your life. A sedentary lifestyle also reduces cardiac output, meaning less blood is pumped by your heart and so less oxygen and nutrients are carried to your brain and organs. More oxygen in your blood means that your muscles get what they need to function efficiently and avoid lactic acid buildup. When you avoid lactic acid buildup, you experience less tiredness and fatigue, which results in feeling healthier and stronger. Things like cellulite, increased body fat, the gradual decrease of lean muscle mass, less energy, and more tiredness have absolutely nothing to do with the natural process of getting older. These aren't symptoms of aging—they are symptoms of a body not working as well as it once did, primarily because the system has been dragged down due to a lack of important nutrients and regular exposure to toxins. It all works together.

Lack of exercise eventually leads to high blood pressure, a weaker heart, and a decline in hormone production, which results in shrinking muscles, thinning bones, a weaker immune system, and a growing inability to concentrate. See the cascade? Like dominoes, one after another the problems of aging—sickness and obesity—begin. But the good news is, it's reversible if you start now.

Regular use of free weights stimulates bone growth, builds lean muscle mass, and creates a cut, defined look that is beautiful. Most women hate their arms. What a drag it is that from middle age on we often have to cover up winter and summer to hide arms that no longer have tone. The tragedy of being sedentary is that without exercise, by the time people are ready to start enjoying their lives they've lost so much lean muscle and aerobic capacity and are so tired and weak they don't feel like doing anything. You see it all the time—older people who are out of gas. Lean muscle mass begins to decline steadily after age thirty. Unless you take steps to stop that decline, by age sixty-five you will have lost 25 percent to 30 percent (or more) of the lean muscle mass and strength you had in your twenties. But again, the good news is this decline can be avoided through exercise.

You don't have to be a fanatic. You don't have to spend hours at the gym. I have laid out what I feel is a good program for losing weight and restoring definition and shape to your body. Age has nothing to do with being strong and fit. In fact, one summer in St. Tropez, our eighty-year-old host, a fitness advocate, towed our small boat into shore (with three full-grown adults inside) holding its rope with one arm while he swam. He was hardly winded when we reached shore. I know it is possible to achieve what you think now is impossible.

GO AHEAD, HAVE A FIT

There are three main components of physical fitness: flexibility, aerobic (cardiovascular conditioning), and strength. How do you get more of each?

Flexibility

I know of no better way to stay flexible than to regularly do yoga. And staying supple is desirable for both women and men. Most every city has a yoga class somewhere; in fact, most anywhere in the world you can find a class. When I was in China, I went to a local yoga class in Shanghai and had a great experience.

Yoga helps me as a writer because after I do my initial workout in the morning I sometimes sit in front of my computer for hours at a time. Anyone familiar with yoga knows the position Pigeon, and it is one of the positions I work into before I go to bed at night. It loosens up my back, so I never have back problems. I originally started yoga because I watched my cat, Gloria, stretch slowly and deliberately each morning, and I realized that I wanted to be as limber and flexible as she was. Yoga is meditative and calming, and you can get a good cardio workout and a great stretch and pull of the muscles. It makes for a long, lean, beautifully toned body. It is something I will do until I die, and that is the beauty of it—you are never too young and never too old. In fact, my four-year-old grandson does yoga in school daily.

If you do not want to do yoga, a Pilates class might appeal to you. If classes just aren't for you, make sure you do some stretching exercises every day.

Aerobic (Cardiovascular Conditioning)

Aerobic exercise increases lung capacity, which gives better-oxygenated blood with every breath you take. Life is air and water (hydration and oxygenation)—they must flow in and out of the cells and are carried to the cells through the bloodstream. Well-oxygenated blood means higher energy, faster healing, stronger immunity, greater endurance, and overall better health, including lower blood pressure, lower triglycerides, and lower LDL cholesterol.

A sedentary lifestyle means less blood is pumped by your heart, which results in less oxygen and nutrients getting to your brain and organs. To compensate for less oxygen and nutrients, the heart beats harder and blood pressure rises, all in an unsuccessful attempt to feed the brain. In other words, the more you move, the healthier you become.

Your body is made for movement. You need a certain amount of physical activity to stay healthy. Without exercise, you become weak from the inside out. More exercise means more energy, improved lung capacity, and more oxygen in your blood; oxygen-rich blood feeds your muscles and your brain to make everything function more efficiently.

Aerobic exercise strengthens your heart and lungs and builds strength and vitality throughout your entire body. Aerobic exercise, or cardio as many are calling it now, can be anything that appeals to you. It doesn't matter how you get your heart beating; just get it beating rapidly at least once a day. Perhaps it's the StairMaster or the elliptical trainer. Or if you have stairs in your house, go up and down them as many times as you can without stopping, adding to the amount of reps as you progress. Other ways to get aerobic exercise could be walking, jogging, cycling, swimming, rebounding (using a mini trampoline), or aerobic classes. If you walk every day, try to walk a little faster and a little farther each time. If you jog, do the same. All of these activities are wonderfully aerobic and the benefits of regular effort will pay off. Again, whatever you choose, try to push yourself a little farther each day.

Aim for thirty minutes a day three or more times a week of moderate aerobic exercise, to burn calories, speed up your metabolism, increase your energy, and strengthen your immune system. If you've never exercised before you might want to attend a class, or buy a DVD, or go to a health club and buy a few sessions with a personal trainer to get you started.

Push yourself! It's for you and your health, and an extra gift will be weight loss. While aerobic exercise is great for your heart and lungs and builds endurance, it does nothing to prevent the gradual loss of lean muscle mass. Only resistance training can restore or increase muscle mass and the most common form of resistance exercise is weight, or strength, training. So that's next on our list.

Strength Training

This is the most beneficial form of exercise to help keep your hormones working efficiently and your bones strong. Studies show that even people in their seventies and eighties can regain and maintain much of their youthful strength simply by doing regular exercise. The most common form of resistance exercise is weight training, although I am quite partial to the EZ Gym (I will say, unabashedly, it is my product). The EZ Gym has resistance bands that attach easily to any door and is so lightweight and easy to install that I travel with mine. It is not cumbersome, it doesn't overwhelm, and it can do the job. You can start with beginning strength and work your way up; full strength is plenty even for the most avid male workout buff. But you don't have to buy this system of resistance bands— any reputable brand will do, as will free weights.

When at home, I alternate between the EZ Gym and free weights, and I constantly push myself to amp up the resistance as my body becomes ready. As soon as a movement becomes too easy I know I am ready to increase it. At present, I have built up to fifteen-pound weights and I find my arms have become nicely toned. Start with a weight or band that suits you, whether it's two pounds, five pounds, or more, then work your way up.

Dr. Michael Colgan in his book *Hormonal Health* says, "Stress on the bone initiated by physical activity is what triggers the electrochemical spark that activates estrogen and progesterone to interact with various minerals and cause the manufacture of new bone material."

Hormones play an important role in bone strength. Bones are made of osteoclasts and osteoblasts; the former are activated by estrogen and testosterone and the latter are activated by progesterone. One hormone burrows holes and the other fills them; burrowing and filling, that is the bone-making process. Weight training is the engine that stimulates this process. The weight, by pulling the muscle against the bone, causes the muscles to stimulate the bone, thus starting the process that hormones play in bone formation. If muscle stress against the bone is insufficient to cause the electrochemical spark, no new bone material is made and eventually the bones weaken.

COMMIT TO CARING

We sit around all day. We no longer do as much physical work as we once did; we live sedentary lives and we are paying the price. Too many older citizens are in wheelchairs or using walkers as a result of bones that no longer hold them up. Don't allow that to happen.

Make a commitment today to add exercise to your life. Choose a convenient time each day and then, as the slogan goes, just do it. By scheduling a workout into your day, it will happen; otherwise you will find excuses to get out of it. This step is invaluable in the Sexy Forever plan. You are now in this for life—a detoxed, hormonally balanced, fit body, all of which equals health, longevity, and feeling and looking good. It can be yours with a little effort.

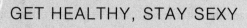

GET HEALTHY, STAY SEXY

THE DAILY MOVES

- Do yoga stretching exercises. If you have never done yoga, attend a class a few times to get the hang of it. I do my own form of yoga, exercising the areas of my body that feel tight and need stretching.

- Work your abdomen. Start with five sit-ups (not crunches—do full sit-ups, the real thing). Then work up to ten and beyond, as many as you can pull off. My Torso Track is great for abs and your upper body. That flabby stomach will disappear in due time. Keep at it. It will happen!

- Work your waist. Lie on the floor with legs bent at the knees. Keep hips flat on the ground and not moving while you bicycle your knees back and forth. Perform fifty, then eventually one hundred daily. This keeps the waist nice and trim.

- Get your heart pumping. Walk briskly for at least a half hour daily. Or go up and down the stairs ten times, working up to twenty times, until it is no longer difficult. And then keep adding, whether it's minutes to your walk or steps to your climb. Or use the elliptical machine or StairMaster at your gym. Just make sure you are breathing hard at the end; you want to get that heart rate up so you can strengthen this most important muscle.

- Work in resistance training two or three times a week. Start with a low weight, perhaps two to five pounds, then work up slowly. You don't want to start with too much poundage or you can injure yourself. A trainer at the gym or health club will be very helpful in designing a weight program for your fitness abilities. Or you can check out my EZ Gym for strength training and no-impact cardio all in one.

After a few weeks of this, start preening in front of the mirror and congratulate yourself on your new healthy, detoxed, hormonally balanced, beautiful, toned body. Life is good!

Step 5

SUPPLEMENT TO SPEED WEIGHT LOSS

Cristiana Paul, M.S., is an independent nutrition consultant in the Los Angeles area and my personal nutritionist. She is an avid reviewer of nutrition research and educates doctors and patients on nutritional therapies and assessments for optimal health. She is also a contributor to the fourth edition of *The Textbook of Natural Medicine*.

Nutrition is the fuel our bodies need to operate. With inferior nutrition our health suffers and we are set up for disease. I asked her how we can stay healthy (and consequently thin) in our toxic environment.

CP: For our bodies to function optimally and efficiently we need to consume a diet balanced with the right amounts of protein, good fat, unrefined carbohydrates, and lots and lots of various forms of fiber (soluble and insoluble). All these aspects are important to maximize fat burning and support body renewal and function.

Most of us need to supplement because we do not get enough nutrients due to poor diet and the deficiency of our soils. The most important supplements are vitamins, minerals, and essential fatty acids, but a few others also play important roles. Relative to weight control, here are some good examples of supplements that may be useful because they are very involved in fat and carbohydrate burning:

Carnitine. This supplement helps fat transport in the mitochondria, where it has a chance to be burned. Carnitine is mostly found in red meat, which many people avoid, and it is also synthesized in the body, but sometimes not enough to support optimal fat burning. A urine test can tell us if we need to supplement. Typical doses are 500 to 1,000 mg/day. It may be especially helpful when taken an hour or two prior to exercise.

Lipoic acid. This plays a role in blood glucose control. If you have elevated or highly fluctuating glucose levels (such as in hypoglycemia) you may consider supplementing with 100 to 1,200 mg (based on a doctor's or nutritionist's evaluation). The bottom line is that lipoic acid will help you burn glucose more efficiently, and in that sense it helps with weight control.

CoQ_{10}. There is a blood test for coenzyme Q_{10} that tells us if we need to supplement. If you take a statin or red yeast rice, the body's production of CoQ_{10} is impaired, so you need to supplement even more. CoQ_{10} is a key factor in energy production and helps us burn fats and carbs more efficiently. In fact, it was shown to help normalize elevated blood glucose in some cases. It also supports heart health and protects the brain. Typical doses are 30 to 100 mg.

Most people are not aware that correcting nutritional deficiencies with a good multivitamin/multimineral and omega-3 supplement will make them much more efficient at burning fat, sugar, and carbohydrates and will also reduce cravings.

Blood and urine testing can help a physician analyze each person's needs for supplementation. At the very minimum you want to take a basic multivitamin/multimineral in a formula that has good absorbable ingredients and no unwanted contaminants. You also want the nutrients to be in a form that they occur in nature if they are available—for example, natural folate (not folic acid), natural mixed tocopherols for vitamin E (not just alpha-tocopherol), natural mixed carotenoids (not just beta-carotene), natural vitamin B_{12} (methylcobalamin or adenosylcobalamin, not cyanocobalamin or hydroxycobalamin), and chelated minerals.

Most people need to supplement with omega-3 fats because their diets provide an excess of omega-6 fats (from cooking oils and animal fats), and it's important to choose fish oil, flaxseed oil, or algae (for vegetarians) that are clean of environmental contaminants (mercury, PCBs) and oxidized fats. Frankly, it is a good idea to ask for a certificate of analysis from the manufacturer for everything you take.

Extracts from green tea were shown in studies to help boost weight loss. It probably does this through a few complementary actions: it boosts the metabolic rate (an increase of 4 percent per twenty-four hours when taking an extract of 370 mg ECGC per day) and it keeps adrenaline elevated longer than normal (which helps fat release from body stores and may reduce hunger). More sustained adrenaline levels may help a person feel more energetic, and he or she may be more likely to exercise or do something physical. For a person with excess adrenaline production (or who has a difficult time breaking it down, such as those with COMT mutations) green tea may increase adrenaline levels to an unhealthy range. On the other hand, for people who are tired all the time because their adrenal glands do not produce adequate amounts of adrenaline, green tea may be helpful. You can drink it or take extracts that contain the equivalent of 2 to 3 cups of green tea in a pill (for example 500 mg ECGC). Also, keep in mind that the body needs tyrosine (an amino acid found in proteins) to make adrenaline. Supplementing with tyrosine (1 to 2 g/day) may boost production of adrenaline and work synergistically with green tea. Too much adrenaline at night is not good, so it's important to make sure that supplements are not affecting your sleep quality. Poor sleep leads to weight gain and health problems, and this effect can be increased by the addition of coffee.

Fiber is important, so try to get 35 to 50 g of fiber daily from both soluble and insoluble forms (read the label, it will tell you). Variety is important with fiber, and avoiding the artificial colors and sweeteners added to most commercial brands is also important. I like Designs for Health PaleoFiber formula because it is a combination of twelve types of fiber from fruits, seeds, gums, vegetables, and roots, and it is gluten, soy, and grain free, so it is most likely hypoallergenic.

Fiber will keep you full longer and help you eat less. It slows down the absorption of sugar, thus reducing insulin production in response to meals. Keep in mind that insulin influences the fat cells to reduce the release of their fat content and also slows down certain fat-burning enzymes. This is not because insulin is an evil hormone but because it is supposed to signal that the body has plenty of glucose, telling it: "Burn the glucose first and save the fat from body storages for later." So you see, if you eat excess carbohydrates and sugar all day long, you impair your ability to tap into your fat stores. (See the Resources for good sources of fiber supplements.)

Fiber also reduces fat and cholesterol and sugar absorption, and it may lower blood levels of cholesterol and triglycerides. Fiber helps detoxify, supports regular bowel movements, and reduces risks of many cancers. I cannot speak enough about the fiber benefits for weight control and health.

In addition to Cristiana's recommendations, I have been looking for supplements from nature that can speed up and enhance your ability to lose weight. And that's what this fifth step is all about: accelerating your results, naturally. With the help of top bioscientists, I've discovered a supplement that does just that.

We've already discussed detoxification and the critical need to release toxins in order to lose fat. We now also know that hormones need to be balanced if there is any hope of losing the weight we put on starting at age forty. You picked up this book to lose weight and this will happen as your body slowly releases the toxins it has accumulated over a lifetime and also when the inflammatory fires created by your food sensitivities quiet down. Now you need to add in the supplements that nature has provided for optimal health, weight control, and the nutrition that has been lost in our food supply.

The good news is that out of the hundreds of nutrients that claim weight loss effects, four have demonstrated weight loss and waist circumference reduction in peer-reviewed scientific studies. This is a science-based product and when I read about the incredible results, all from natural ingredients, I knew I had to make the results available to everyone.

The Sexy Forever Weight Loss Formula includes:

1. LuraLean

2. *Phaseolus vulgaris*

3. Irvingia

4. Green tea phytosome

LuraLean

This ingredient helps control the absorption of some calories if taken before the two heaviest meals of the day. By maintaining its viscous structure throughout the digestive tract, LuraLean is able to stop the absorption of ingested fats and carbohydrates. LuraLean is a fiber composed of specially processed glucomannan—a water-soluble polysaccharide derived from a tuberous plant that grows only in the remote mountains of northern Japan.

This translates into weight reduction. One clinical study showed that without any dietary changes (participants ate and drank whatever they wanted), those taking LuraLean lost 5.5 pounds after eight weeks compared to a 1.5-pound weight gain in the placebo group. In a similar study, those taking LuraLean (twice a day before breakfast and dinner) lost 7.04 pounds compared to a gain of almost 1 pound in the placebo arm of the study. These studies showed substantial reductions in blood triglycerides, cholesterol, and LDL (bad cholesterol) levels in the LuraLean groups compared to increases in these dangerous blood fats in the placebo arms.

Looking at the blood test results of typical healthy twenty-one-year-olds, scientists noticed that they had very low levels of blood glucose, cholesterol, and triglycerides. Even if people do not change their diet, by the time they reach age fifty their blood glucose, triglycerides, and cholesterol are usually much higher. Fifty-year-olds typically weigh more than when they were twenty-one, especially in the abdominal region of their bodies. There are correlations between blood glucose and triglyceride levels and unwanted weight gain. To put it simply, the same calories a twenty-one-year-old can safely ingest become increasingly toxic as we age. This is because aging causes us to lose the metabolic capacity to utilize ingested calories in efficient energy-expending ways. Not only do these calories induce body fat storage, but they also increase vascular disease risks. That is why taking LuraLean before the two heaviest meals of the day is so important. It helps impede absorption of excess sugars and fats in your diet, while helping to reduce the amount of food you consume with each meal.

Phaseolus vulgaris

Researchers at the UCLA School of Medicine have successfully used extracts from the white kidney bean (*Phaseolus vulgaris*) to target alpha-amylase. A study was done where thirty obese adults took either a placebo or the *Phaseolus vulgaris* extract. After eight weeks, those taking the white bean extract lost 3.8 pounds in weight, and more important, 1.5 inches of abdominal fat. The group taking the *Phaseolus vulgaris* also had a three-fold reduction in triglyceride levels compared with the placebo group, which helps corroborate the role of weight loss and simultaneous reduction in artery-clogging triglyceride levels.

Another more impressive study of *Phaseolus vulgaris* showed that those who consumed the most carbohydrates lost the most weight. In this study, subjects who supplemented with *Phaseolus vulgaris* and consumed the highest levels of dietary starch lost 8.7 pounds compared with only 1.7 pounds in the control group over four weeks. Even more impressive was the 3.3 inches of belly fat lost in the *Phaseolus vulgaris* group versus only 1.3 inches in the controls. In a double-blind study on sixty overweight volunteers, half the study participants received *Phaseolus vulgaris* while the other half were given a placebo. Both groups were placed on a 2,000–2,200-calorie diet. After only thirty days, those taking *Phaseolus vulgaris* lost 6.5 pounds of weight and 1.2 inches in waist size compared with 0.8 pounds and 0.2 inches in the placebo group.

As we age, it becomes increasingly difficult to keep belly fat off. At the same time, we are challenged to keep blood glucose levels in optimal ranges. The exploding rates of type 2 diabetes and obesity are a testament to the dual problem of weight gain caused by the absorption of too many calories from simple carbohydrates.

Irvingia

Irvingia is a West African plant extract (from *Irvingia gabonesis*) that has been shown to help support leptin sensitivity in overweight people. Fat cells (called adipocytes) secrete leptin, a hormone that tells your brain you've eaten enough. Leptin also helps with the breakdown of stored (triglyceride) fat in our fat cells. Overweight people have higher blood levels of leptin, indicating that their cells have become resistant to leptin. In a published study, irvingia demonstrated beneficial effects on leptin blood levels, followed by a weight loss of over 20 pounds on average in ten weeks and an average reduction in waist circumference of about 6 inches. Study subjects taking irvingia reported consuming fewer calories, which makes sense, based on the enhanced leptin sensitivity brought about by this plant extract. Irvingia also has alpha-amylase-inhibiting properties similar to *Phaseolus vulgaris*. Inhibiting amylase helps slow the rate of carbohydrate absorption, reducing the caloric impact of starchy and sugary foods.

Large meals overload the bloodstream with calories and later cause a rebound increase in appetite when blood sugar levels plummet in response to excess release of insulin. One way of stopping this after-meal glucose-insulin rebound is to take nutrients that neutralize the carbohydrate-degrading enzyme alpha-amylase before meals.

Scientific data suggests that irvingia also helps support healthy adiponectin levels. Adiponectin is a hormone that helps maintain the insulin sensitivity of our energy-producing cells. Large fat cells found in overweight people produce less adiponectin. This means that these individuals need to be concerned about maintaining enough adiponectin to support insulin sensitivity, something that we lose during normal aging.

Most people don't know this, but the majority of body fat consists of triglycerides that are stored in our fat cells. A reason that weight loss and triglyceride reduction go hand in hand is that triglycerides make up the bulk of our fat storage. We get triglycerides directly from the fat we eat, and also from the conversion of excess glucose in our blood to triglycerides stored in our fat cells. In the latter instance, glucose is converted to triglycerides by an enzyme called glycerol-3-phosphate dehydrogenase. Irvingia inhibits glycerol-3-phosphate dehydrogenase, reducing the amount of ingested sugars that are converted to body fat.

Green tea phytosome

We all know about the great benefits of green tea. Aging robs us of the ability to efficiently burn fat as energy. Instead we store fat in our adipocytes (fat cells). The components responsible for green tea's weight loss benefits are polyphenol compounds that increase metabolic energy expenditure and hence calorie burning. The problem is getting enough of green tea's polyphenols absorbed into the blood. But a group of Italian researchers created a proprietary green tea phytosome that increased the polyphenols' ability to be absorbed into the bloodstream. In a human clinical trial using this green tea phytosome, the weight loss effects were substantial. This study involved one hundred overweight subjects, half of whom received the green tea phytosome. Both groups were placed on reduced-calorie diets (approximately 1,850 calories/day for men and 1,350 calories/day for women).

After ninety days on the reduced-calorie diet, the control group lost 9.9 pounds. The group taking the green tea phytosome, on the other hand, lost a whopping 30.1 pounds—more than triple the weight loss of the control group! There was a 10 percent reduction in the green tea phytosome group's belly size compared with a 5 percent reduction in the control group. Male participants did even better in this category, showing a 14 percent reduction in waist circumference compared with a 7 percent reduction in the control group.

What's so interesting about this study is that it shows that people can lose considerable weight (9.9. pounds) by eating fewer calories. Yet when this green tea phytosome was added, the total amount of weight lost tripled (to 30.1 pounds) while twice as much belly fat disappeared. Scientists attribute these remarkable benefits to the ability of green tea to boost resting metabolic rates and reduce the absorption of dietary fats, which makes this green tea phytosome an ideal nutrient to take before heavy meals.

If you are going to turn your life around by eliminating toxic foods, as discussed in this book, adding these four supplements can boost your ability to lose weight more quickly and safely, with no drugs or stimulants.

Each one of these weight loss tools was developed in a different part of the world, subjected to controlled scientific study, and some were even awarded patent status by the U.S. Patent and Trademark office.

I have manufactured all four of these supplements into just one formula. The Sexy Forever Weight Loss Formula is available at Suzanne Somers.com. Click on Sexy Forever for a list of all of my products.

THE IMPORTANCE OF MINERALS IN GETTING HEALTHY—AND GETTING TO A HEALTHY WEIGHT

Minerals are essential to life, but today it is very difficult to get them through food alone. There are just less of them in our natural food supply. Not only that—because people are eating processed food in quantities never before experienced, these vital minerals are absent from that food, too. This deficiency is a big contributor to the problems of obesity, fatigue, and heart disease.

The minerals that are most missing in today's food supply are selenium, zinc, manganese, potassium, iron, magnesium, copper, boron, and chromium. Here's what you need to know about them—and how to get more of them each day:

- Selenium is an antioxidant that slows the aging process and helps maintain a youthful elasticity in your tissues. It helps hot flashes and menopausal stress. It strengthens the immune system, pancreas, and liver.

- Zinc is vital to maintaining enzyme systems (crucial for cancer protection) and is essential for protein synthesis. Zinc helps in the formulation of insulin, normalizes the prostate, and is important for brain function. Signs of zinc deficiency include amnesia, apathy, brittle nails, depression, diarrhea, fatigue, hair loss, a weak immune system, irritability, lethargy, loss of appetite, loss of sense of taste, memory impairment, difficulty seeing at night, impaired wound healing, and more.

- Manganese helps activate the enzymes necessary for your body to properly utilize vitamin B_1 and vitamin C. It is used in the formation of thyroxine, which is the principal hormone of the thyroid gland, and it plays an important role in the digestive and nervous systems. The proper balance of manganese eliminates fatigue, improves memory, and reduces irritability.

- Potassium works with sodium to regulate your body's water balance and normalize heart rhythms. Nerve and muscle function suffer if the sodium-potassium balance is off. Insufficient potassium can lead to mental and physical distress. Potassium aids in clearer thinking by sending oxygen to your brain, and it also helps dispose of body waste. It is an important factor in helping to reduce high blood pressure and in fighting allergies.

- Iron is not for everyone. But for those who require iron, it is critical to the oxygenation of the blood and is used in producing hormones and prostaglandins that affect blood, muscles, and enzymes in your body. Symptoms of iron deficiency are anemia, brittle nails, confusion, constipation, depression, dizziness, fatigue, headaches, oral lesions, and many more. Iron supplements should be taken only if your blood tests show a deficiency. Too much iron is not good, especially in men.

- Magnesium is necessary for calcium and vitamin C metabolism. It is essential for effective nerve and muscle functioning and converting blood sugar into energy. It fights stress and depression, promotes heart health, keeps teeth whiter, and prevents calcium deposits, kidney stones, and gallstones. When taken with calcium it acts as a natural tranquilizer. Symptoms of deficiency include anxiety, confusion, heart problems, hyperactivity, insomnia, nervousness, muscular irritability, restlessness, and weakness. As many as 75 to 85 percent of Americans are magnesium deficient.

- Copper plays an essential role in converting your body's iron into hemoglobin. It activates certain amino acids (essential to life) and is important in the body's utilization of vitamin C. Symptoms of copper deficiency include anemia, arterial damage, depression, fatigue, fragile bones, hair loss, and others. American diets are estimated to be deficient in copper by as much as 75 percent.

- Boron is a helper mineral that works in conjunction with, and increases the effectiveness of, several other minerals.

- Chromium works with insulin in the metabolism of sugar and, as such, works as a nutritional deterrent to type 2 diabetes.

All of the above minerals are available in one-packet form. Go to SuzanneSomers.com and click on Sexy Forever for information on how to order them.

GOODBYE INFLAMMATION, GOODBYE EXCESS FAT

Our toxic diets set the stage for a chronic inflammatory condition that not only damages the body's tissues, but also precludes successful weight loss. When we have too many fat cells, the result is an excess release of inflammatory factors that interfere with our ability to shed fat pounds. Fat cells (especially in the abdominal region) secrete pro-inflammatory chemicals that are carried to the liver, where C-reactive protein is formed. As you accumulate more body fat, C-reactive protein blood levels rise. You may have heard that elevated levels of C-reactive protein are associated with heart attack and stroke risk. What you may not have read about is the impact that C-reactive protein has in promoting excess fat storage. Leptin and insulin are two fat regulators in the body. Elevated C-reactive protein interferes with the ability of insulin to utilize glucose. Excess C-reactive protein also interferes with the ability of leptin to control appetite and burn fat. As we gain more fat pounds, the ability of leptin and insulin to regulate our body weight is impaired because fat cells secrete chemical messengers that stimulate the formation of C-reactive protein.

By following the steps you have learned about so far in this book, your C-reactive protein levels should start to decline as you slowly shed extra fat and pounds. Also, as discussed, restoring a youthful hormone balance can lower pro-inflammatory chemicals in the blood. Unfortunately, the aging process itself increases C-reactive protein levels, making it necessary to take steps to prevent chronic inflammation from sabotaging our health.

Food cooked at high temperatures promotes inflammation in the body—something we don't want to happen when trying to lose weight. Just changing how your foods are prepared can help you shed body fat.

One of the most important nutrients to obtain in your diet are omega-3 fatty acids, which help reduce C-reactive protein but also activate our mitochondria (the energy centers of our cells) to burn dietary fats. If you increase your intake of omega-3s from cold-water fish (especially wild salmon), walnuts, and flaxseed, and at the same time reduce omega-6 fats from corn, sunflower, safflower, and other vegetable oils, you will have taken an important step in getting healthy and thin again.

It's difficult to get enough omega-3s from your diet. I take a purified fish oil supplement that provides the following minimum in each daily dose: 1,400 mg of EPA, 1,000 mg of DHA, and 20 mg of sesame lignan extract. Research suggests that sesame lignans, in combination with fish oil, synergistically support the metabolism of fatty acids in the liver—this means the effect is more than additive! The failure of the liver to properly metabolize fatty acids can result in excess accumulation of triglycerides. And triglycerides that are not metabolized accumulate and contribute to weight gain.

When rats were fed sesame lignans and fish oil together, their liver fatty acid oxidation rates rose much higher than when fed fish oil alone. This study pointed out that the combination of sesame and fish oil worked synergistically by increasing the fatty acid oxidation enzymes in the liver. The combination of fish oil and sesame can improve mitochondrial fatty acid energy utilization, which facilitates triglyceride reduction—an important step in shedding fat pounds.

In conventional medicine the big concern is cholesterol. Yet in the alternative world, inflammation is the larger issue. Chronic inflammation is an indicator of a present problem or the makings of one. Chronic inflammation can be determined by taking a blood test called highly sensitive C-reactive protein (for information on how to get this blood test see Resources). C-reactive protein interferes with the ability of leptin to regulate fat storage in the body. Consuming more omega-3s, cutting back on omega-6 fats and foods cooked at high temperatures, and eliminating sugary (high-glycemic) foods will help suppress the inflammatory fires that rage in the bodies of overweight people.

GET HEALTHY, STAY SEXY

In addition to the list of weight loss products I reference at the beginning of the chapter, here is a more expansive list of supplements I take each day. This amount may be too overwhelming to some, but I believe this antiaging cocktail will lower your C-reactive protein, increase your ability to lose weight, and build your immune system.

NUTRIENT	DAILY DOSE	WHAT YOU NEED TO KNOW
Curcumin	400 mg	Use only specialized forms of curcumin documented to fully absorb into the bloodstream.
R-lipoic acid	150–300 mg	Don't confuse R-lipoic acid with cheaper alpha-lipoic acid supplements. R-lipoic acid is twice as potent.
Carnitine	2,000 mg	Use only acetyl-L-carnitine, glycine propionyl-L-carnitine, and/or acetyl-L-carnitine arginate, as these forms are better utilized.

Coenzyme Q$_{10}$	100–200 mg	Use only the ubiquinol form of CoQ$_{10}$, as it is much better absorbed into the bloodstream than conventional ubiquinone.
Gamma-linolenic acid (GLA)	200–600 mg	Make sure 10 mg of sesame lignans are included with each capsule to facilitate formation of a powerful anti-inflammatory substance called prostaglandin E1.
Resveratrol	250 mg	Make sure your supplement label states you are getting 250 mg of trans-resveratrol. Ideally it should be combined with pterostilbene and quercetin for optimal results.
Magnesium	500 mg	Take with food to minimize the potential for diarrhea.
Vitamin E	200 mg	Make sure to take at least 200 mg of the gamma-tocopherol form of vitamin E in addition to the alpha-tocopherol form found in your multivitamin.

Vitamin D	5,000 IU	Most multivitamins contain only 400 IU of vitamin D. New studies show this is woefully inadequate to regulate inflammatory factors in the body.
Vitamin K_2	100 mcg	This anti-inflammatory nutrient is deficient in many people. Make sure that your vitamin K contains 100 mcg of the MK-7 form of vitamin K along with vitamin K_1.
EPA/DHA	2,400 mg	If you choose to get EPA and DHA (omega-3s) from fish oil, make sure the fish oil has been purified to remove contaminants.

PART III

The Eating Plan and Recipes

THE THREE-PHASE
WEIGHT LOSS PLAN

Now that you understand how you have arrived at your current state of health, you can take the necessary steps to improve your life by detoxifying your body and restoring it with proper nutrition, and in the process find your ideal body weight. I know good health should always be the motivation for how we live our lives, but let's face it—many of us really decide to get on top of our health only when we don't like the way we look. It's shallow, and I am just as guilty when it comes to vanity, but I've now embraced good health and quality of life as key goals. It used to be easier, and when I think back on my past, during the periods when I was slim and looking good, I realize I used to eat and drink anything and everything, no matter its health consequences. I paid a big price. I would freely eat pasta with cream sauce, drink as much wine as I wanted, and the desserts—oh, my sweet tooth! It wasn't until I gained some weight that I really cared about what I was eating. Of course, cancer changed all of that for me. It made me recommit to my health in a way that would keep me on course for life.

In this chapter, we take all the general steps you've learned to date in the book and apply them in the Sexy Forever three-phase action plan:

- DETOX PHASE: Days 1 to 30

- LEVEL 1—WEIGHT LOSS PHASE: Days 31 through reaching your goal weight

- LEVEL 2—LIFESTYLE PHASE: Maintaining your weight and health for the rest of your life

All readers should start with the Detox Phase. In the Detox Phase, you will clean out your pantry and fridge. In addition, I ask you to stay within fairly strict guidelines for your daily meals. What you will love about this phase is that you will see results quickly! But it's not just fat you are losing—you are eliminating toxins stored within the fat, with the goal of a clean, healthy system that is working at its peak.

After the Detox Phase, you start the Weight Loss Phase. During this time you will eat within the outlined nutrition guidelines, which comprise a variety of proteins, healthy fats, whole-grain carbohydrates, lots of fresh vegetables, and fruit. You will continue to avoid sugar, chemicals, processed foods, and alcohol.

Once you reach your goal weight, you will live the Level 2—Lifestyle Phase, a simple plan to maintain your weight and good health forever. When you find your ideal weight and your body is detoxed from the chemical onslaught, you'll learn here how to make everyday choices to continue this lifestyle for the long, healthy road ahead of you.

This goal is within your reach. This new body is yours for the taking. This level of optimum health is achievable! Let's get started.

GETTING SEXY FOREVER

Those of you who are familiar with my Somersize program will recognize the basic tenets of the Sexy Forever nutrition plan. As always, I upgrade and improve my philosophies based upon the new knowledge I gain from the experts I am fortunate to have constantly feeding me information. Even more importantly, I learn from *you* and the experiences you pass along to me at SuzanneSomers.com, on my Facebook page, and at SexyForeverPlan.com/book.

Many of the millions who have used my weight loss plan understand that to truly change your lifestyle, you must eliminate processed foods and retrain yourself to eat the foods you find at the perimeter of the grocery store—fresh produce, healthy fats, clean protein, and whole grains. If you adopt this notion, you will see most of the other questions you have will answer themselves. That being said, I am barraged with questions like this: "I have a bottle of salad dressing that contains guar gum, sucralose, and modified food starch . . . is that okay to eat?" In most cases, if you ask, you already know the answer. While some of these products may technically comply with the guidelines of my weight loss program, you are always better off avoiding packaged, bottled, or processed foods with preservatives, chemicals, and fillers. The Sexy Forever plan embraces this commitment to clean, real food at a new level. I have always recommended eating real food, but the damaging effects of the alternatives are now clearer than ever to me.

At the back of the book you will find a Food Reference Guide suitable for each phase, as well as things to avoid.

SEXY FOREVER: THE BASICS

1. Eliminate Insulin Triggers (foods that raise insulin levels: sugar, refined grains, starchy vegetables, and alcohol) and bad fats (such as trans fats).

2. Commit to clean, real organic food. Eliminate chemicals, toxins, fillers, and preservatives. Eat organic whenever possible.

3. Combine Proteins with Healthy Fats and Vegetables. Eat from the Sexy Forever list of Proteins and Healthy Fats, in combination with Vegetables (low-starch).

4. Watch those Carbohydrates. Eat approved, nutrient-rich Carbohy-
    drates, in specific portion sizes, at select meals.

5. Eat Fruit on an empty stomach, to maximize digestion and nutrient
    absorption.

6. Eat three meals per day. To increase metabolism, you must not skip
    meals.

7. Hydrate. Drink eight 8-ounce glasses of water each day.

8. Wait two hours between meals or snacks if switching from a Carbo-
    hydrate to a Protein/Healthy Fats meal or vice versa.

Eliminate Insulin Triggers

To succeed in detoxifying your system, you need to start by cleaning out
the fridge and the pantry. The first foods you need to eliminate are the
ones that trigger a large insulin response; these are foods that are high in
sugar or starch. This knocks out obvious foods, like cakes, cookies, candy,
pies, muffins, and pasta or bread made with white flour, and it also includes foods with hidden sugars, like carrots, corn, potatoes, and bananas.
Why is this essential to losing weight? When you eat sugars or high-starch
foods, your blood sugar rises. It is then the job of the pancreas to release
insulin, a hormone responsible for balancing blood sugar. When we are
young and everything is working optimally, we eat sugar, then insulin is
released to balance the blood sugar, and the sugar is burned off as fuel.
As we age, problems arise when our systems can no longer process the
amount of sugar or starches we are regularly ingesting.

Let's recap what we learned about insulin earlier. The reason insulin is
called the fat-storing hormone is that it is solely responsible for deciding if the
sugar you eat is needed for energy or if it should be stored as fat for later use.
If you don't need energy, the insulin will place that sugar into your fat cells,
particularly those around the midsection. If you are thick through the middle, it's probably because you are ingesting too many sugars and starches.

Since insulin is such an important factor in deciding if food is burned off as fuel or stored as fat, a major part of the plan is controlling our insulin levels. What happens when you eliminate Insulin Triggers (sugars and starches) from your diet? When your body needs an energy source, it first looks to the food you eat. If there are no quick forms of energy, such as sugar and white flour, your body will need to look for the next available supply of energy—your stored fat! Your body will then rely upon burning off your stored fat to fuel itself with energy. And unlike the ups and downs in energy you get from eating sugar and processed foods, your fat reserves supply a steady source of slow-burning energy. This is how we supercharge your metabolism and transform you from a carb-burning machine into a fat-burning one.

Insulin Triggers are those foods that have the most detrimental effect on blood sugar levels, and are easily determined by looking at the food's glycemic index. (Lists of the glycemic index of various foods can be found online at SexyForever.com/book.) For example, beer ranks higher on the list than pure sugar—meaning it is absorbed very quickly into the bloodstream, causing a spike in blood sugar and a subsequent spike in insulin. Now it should be pretty clear why those who drink too much beer end up with a beer belly! Other foods high on the list include sugar, white flour, honey, carrots, potatoes, and bananas.

The Food Reference Guide contains a list of Insulin Triggers to eliminate. The big ones are sugars (sugar, corn syrup, honey, etc.), white flour (white bread, white pasta), white rice, high-starch vegetables (potatoes, corn), high-starch fruit (bananas), and alcohol. (Sorry! I know you love that white wine. Me too. Sigh!) For the Detox Phase, you will avoid these foods completely. No worries—we have all-natural sweeteners to replace sugar, and you will learn to love whole grains in place of the white-flour breads and pastas. During the Level 1—Weight Loss Phase, I have substitutes for these foods that will make you feel like you are cheating, but you will continue eating low-glycemic-index foods to release all that stored energy in your fat cells. Once all the stored sugar is cleaned out of your cells and you have reached your ideal body weight, you will enter Level 2—Lifestyle Phase. This is how you will live healthfully for the remainder of your days—even while you splurge on select special occasions.

DIABETES, A ONE-TWO PUNCH

Diabetes is a huge problem in this country, with tens of millions of sufferers (and millions more who have no idea they have it). Many people are confused by this condition and what the difference is between type 1 and type 2 diabetes. It's important to understand the causes of each, so you can take the best, appropriate steps for safeguarding your health.

Type 1 diabetes is a genetically preconditioned disease, usually considered autoimmune in origin, where a person does not make enough insulin; when that person eats sugar, this lack of insulin response does not allow the cells to absorb that sugar. *Type 2 diabetes* is a condition that develops over time due to poor eating habits. It used to be called adult-onset diabetes, but in the past few decades so many children have developed it, they had to alter the name. This increase is due to the shocking decline of nutrition in our diets that has led to rampant obesity and the health-related diseases that come with it. Sadly, this condition continues plaguing the citizens of our country at younger and younger ages.

Type 2 diabetes starts with insulin resistance. Normally, if we eat sugar or carbs and don't need them for immediate energy, insulin signals the cells to store glucose for future use. But with insulin resistance, the cells don't respond normally to insulin and glucose can't enter the cells as easily. Blood glucose levels remain high, and the pancreas keeps producing insulin in a continuing effort to store the sugar. When insulin resistance is very high, there is plenty of insulin available, but it can't do its job of moving blood sugar into cells, so both the insulin and the blood sugar are high. This stage is called type 2 diabetes. In time, this process wears out the pancreas and insulin production slows or even stops. If insulin production stops, this is also called type 1 diabetes—as there is no insulin—but it comes from exhaustion of the cells which make insulin, not from an autoimmune process.

Insulin resistance is the true enemy when it comes to numerous health problems, including high blood pressure, high levels of triglycerides, poor cholesterol levels, chronic inflammation, increased risk of heart disease, and some forms of cancer. Numerous studies document the correlation of high insulin levels with these diseases, yet many people are still more worried about eating a steak or a dollop of sour cream than they are with eating chemically processed, sugary foods that send your insulin levels soaring. *Fat is not the enemy!* Sugar, starches, and the other insulin triggers are the foods you should be most concerned about limiting.

Now you understand why it is vitally important to eliminate Insulin Triggers to improve your health and keep your metabolism burning on high. Take a look at every food in your house; carefully check the ingredient lists. If it contains any form of sugar, white flour, or any of the foods on the Insulin Triggers list (page 291), it needs to be removed from your diet. Rid your pantry and your refrigerator of these foods, including sodas, candy, crackers, white pasta, white bread, poor-quality protein bars, chips, and more.

Don't worry—you will look and feel sooooo good, it will all be worth it. The Sexy Forever plan will teach you the habits we all should have been raised with to enjoy good nutrition for life. Use this opportunity to create a new lifestyle that creates radiantly good health for you and your family. You may not have had the information before . . . but now, no more excuses! Take this chance to change your life.

Eliminate Unhealthy Fats

In addition to high-glycemic-index foods, we will eliminate unhealthy fats. As I have mentioned, the worst offenders are trans fats. Trans fats come mostly from partially hydrogenated oil, which changes the structure of the oil to make it solid and make products that contain it more shelf-stable. Trans fats are the worst type of fat. All those products that claim to taste like butter but are not actually butter—trash them and get the real thing.

I have commented at length about the importance of omega-3 fatty acids. The best oils to include in your diet are olive, perilla, flaxseed, and

fish oils. In addition to trans fats, eliminate corn, cottonseed, peanut, safflower, sunflower, and vegetable oils.

Commit to Clean, Real, Organic Food

You know how I feel about this. Now it is your turn to make a commitment to selecting the highest-quality food you can find. I know how
expensive it is to eat this way. Do what you can, and where you do not
have access or cannot afford these products, use the tricks outlined in the
previous chapters to avoid the worst offenders.

And by all means, make some noise! Demand more organic products at
your store. If we demand more organic foods, the prices will eventually
come down. We must start somewhere. Demand information on the protein sources you purchase—are meats grass-fed? Remember, we do not
want corn-fed protein! Ask about your fish—is it farmed? Insist on wild-
caught selections. Fruits and vegetables—find nearby farmer's markets,
or plant some seeds in the backyard or in a pot garden and grow a few of
your own fruits and vegetables. Yes, it's an effort; it's also *your life*.

Sprays, pesticides, poor-quality protein sources, chemical fillers, preservatives, genetically modified foods, and artificial sweeteners all add to our
toxic burden. *Sexy Forever* will help you release that toxic burden so you
can finally lose the weight and get healthy. Once you get your system
cleaned out, do your best to avoid those foods and conditions that created
this unhealthy environment in the first place.

You will find a complete list of toxins to eliminate in the Food Reference Guide (page 291). Some get overwhelmed by the list and put on
blinders. Every choice you make to ingest one less chemical is a step in
the right direction. Do what you can! Again, you want to do your best
here, knowing none of us can possibly eliminate all the toxins we come
across each day.

Combine Protein, Healthy Fats, and Vegetables

In the Food Reference Guide, you will see I have clearly divided real,
healthy, nutritious foods into the following categories: Protein, Healthy
Fats, Carbohydrates, Vegetables, and Fruits. These are the foods that nur-

ture our bodies. This is the real food our bodies need to thrive. This is the food that will turn off the overactive hunger signal because the body will have the fuel it needs to work optimally.

At breakfast you may choose to have Carbohydrates or Protein, but at lunch and dinner, you will always start with Protein, then add Healthy Fats, plus lots of fresh low-starch Vegetables. This combination of foods fuels your metabolism. Putting it into action simply means you will start with any of the foods on the Protein list, then add any of the foods on the Healthy Fats list, plus any of the foods on the Vegetables list. For example, start with chicken, cooked in olive oil, and served with broccoli; this type of simple combination of Protein, Healthy Fats, and Vegetables will become the mainstay of your meals. You will learn how to add Carbohydrates along the way, but the foundation is the Protein/Fat/Vegetable combo. (Assistance with meal plans and an extensive selection of recipes are available at SexyForever.com/book.)

Protein

Protein provides essential amino acids; the building blocks needed for most every human function from thinking to walking to breathing. Humans need about 9 grams of protein for every 20 pounds of body weight. (For example, if you weigh 160 pounds, you'd need to consume about 72 grams of protein each day.) I suggest a 6- to 8-ounce serving of protein at each meal. This means that a piece of chicken, meat, or fish about the size of the palm of your hand is what you are aiming for. One of these servings will net you anywhere between 36 and 48 grams of protein, dependent on the source. This will help fill you up and make you feel satisfied. Protein sources include meat, poultry, seafood, eggs, cheese, and more. Again, you will find a list of approved Protein sources in the Food Reference Guide (page 291).

Healthy Fats

Next, add some Healthy Fats. I use olive oil at most meals. I use it to marinate and cook my protein. I sauté my vegetables in it. I drizzle it on my salads. For certain meals, I will use coconut oil, or when I want a neutral taste, grapeseed oil. I also use butter and full-fat dairy products like sour cream. I eat Healthy Fats freely, but I don't go crazy eating sticks of butter just because I can. Fortunately, your body will not allow you to overeat these foods. Unlike with refined carbohydrates—where you can eat bag after bag of chips, crackers, and cookies—eating fats sends a signal to your body that you are satiated. Additional Healthy Fats can be found in the Food Reference Guide (page 291).

Vegetables

The Vegetables in the plan are all low-starch vegetables to supercharge your day with antioxidants and fiber. Broccoli, green beans, asparagus, zucchini, kale, tomatoes, fennel, lettuce, celery, and so many more choices will fill your meals. While there is no limit to how many servings of these vegetables you include, you *must* include at least six servings of vegetables each day. I know it sounds like a lot, but a serving is 1 cup of raw vegetables or greens, or ½ cup cooked. That's really not that much. If you have a big salad for lunch, that's probably four servings right there. Then you have a cup of cooked green beans for dinner and you are there. I eat more than six servings per day, but this is the minimum to make sure you are getting enough natural fiber and antioxidants.

This is a shift from my Somersize guidelines. The reason I am adjusting the program is that I don't want you filling up on proteins and fats with no vegetables. Again, I am retraining you to eat real food, well balanced and in reasonable portions. I found that with Somersize, some people understood the balance of the program and adopted a lifestyle of healthy foods, but others would just eat bacon cheeseburgers and never include a vegetable. While you can lose weight eating only proteins and fats, you must include vegetables for both the essential nutrients and the antioxidant benefits. On the other hand, if you are used to filling up on starches, eating your fill of vegetables will also be a shift for you!

A full list of these Vegetables is in the Food Reference Guide (page 291). My companion site, SexyForever.com/book, provides meal plans that ensure you get the nutrients you need.

Carbohydrates

Once the low-carb movement hit, suddenly we shifted from counting fat grams to obsessively counting every carb in sight! I have never believed in eliminating carbohydrates—it's just that some are much better for you than others. As mentioned, the Sexy Forever plan asks you to eliminate Insulin Triggers (it's all about those hormones), but some of these foods will be brought back, in moderation, as you progress with the phases of the program.

In the Detox Phase (days 1 to 30) we will eliminate all Insulin Triggers (sugar, white flour, potatoes, corn, alcohol, etc.), but we will include moderate amounts of approved Carbohydrates (whole-grain bread, brown rice, beans, nuts, whole-wheat pasta, nonfat dairy products). Once we reach Level 1 we slightly increase the approved Carbohydrates with our meals. For Level 2, you will learn to handle a few of those Insulin Triggers every now and then and see the return of the potato.

The key in adding these approved Carbohydrates is eating them at the right time and in the right quantity. We are a nation that overeats carbohydrates—especially refined carbohydrates. Now you get to eat carbohydrates, but only the good ones.

DETOX PHASE

Up to three servings Carbohydrates per day

> While in the Detox Phase, you will eat up to three servings of Carbs, but you cannot combine them with any fats. You may choose to have all of these servings at breakfast in a Carbohydrate-only meal, or you may have one as a midmorning snack and one as a midafternoon snack.

WEIGHT LOSS PHASE

Up to four servings Carbohydrates per day

> In Level 1, you may have up to four total servings; again, you may eat them alone at breakfast or as a snack, or you may add one serving to a meal with Protein, Healthy Fats, and Vegetables.

When you are adding a serving of Carbohydrate to a Protein/Fat/Vegetable meal, it's important that you don't go crazy on the Fats for that meal. This gives you a little more freedom.

LIFESTYLE PHASE

Carbohydrates at your discretion

During Level 2, you will have even more access to good carbs, now that your cells are cleaned out.

NOTE: If you are gluten intolerant, obviously you will have fewer choices on this list, but you still follow the guidelines, using beans, wild rice, quinoa, and other gluten-free carbohydrates. If you're a little confused, don't worry. This will be clearly laid out for you in the sample meal plans.

For you Somersizers—I realize this is all new information. The purpose for this shift, again, is to condition you to eat properly balanced meals, in proportions that accelerate weight loss and support your body nutritionally. While these approved carbohydrates will produce a small insulin response, I have found adding this small amount of low-glycemic carbohydrates supports serotonin production (one of our feel-good hormones) and helps us to feel satiated. In the past, I recommended you get your carbohydrates from low-starch vegetables, but as I said, people were opting out of eating vegetables at all. Now, as you can see, I've insisted on including vegetables, and I'm giving you the option to include a small portion of approved carbohydrates with meals or snacks.

Your weight loss patterns will help you determine the amount of carbohydrates you include in your daily meal plan. If you are not losing steadily, you may need to back off on the carbs. If you are losing steadily, stay within the serving amounts recommended. Each of us has a different metabolism, and you need to customize the plan to work for you. At SexyForever.com/book, we can customize a program just for you.

Fruit

Fruit contains natural sugar, but it still causes a rise in your blood sugar and a release of insulin. Unlike refined sugars, however, fruit also contains a good source of fiber, which slows the effect of sugar in your bloodstream. Plus it's loaded with nutrition—all those fabulous antioxidants! While some low-carb programs recommend eliminating fruit, there are too many health benefits to be that extreme. Instead, the Sexy Forever plan guides you to eat fruit in a way that maximizes your digestion and allows you to reap the benefits of the vitamins, minerals, fiber, and phytonutrients clinically proven to reduce the risk of cancer, stroke, heart disease, and high blood pressure. Plus, fruit is nature's most amazing sweet!

It's always better to eat whole fruit than to drink fruit juice. The whole fruit provides much more fiber, and remember, that slows the absorption of blood sugar into your body. Fruit juice is very high in natural sugar—especially juices that contain fruit juice concentrate as sweeteners. Similarly, dried fruit is very high in natural sugar. Therefore, it's best to eat whole fresh fruit to avoid those intense surges of insulin and to get all of nature's benefits. Frozen fruit is a great asset in making fruit smoothies, for an icy treat. This is the only place where I will sometimes add a little fruit juice—to make my morning smoothie.

Alan provides a good example to understanding how much natural sugar is found in fruit. He has a serious addiction to fresh fruit. He craves it. Now that I understand his gluten sensitivity, it all makes sense. Because he was fighting a serious allergy to gluten, his body was not absorbing nutrition. This is what made him feel so tired; his body was craving sugar as a means for survival. Whereas with my granddaughter the food intolerance fueled a craving for sugar, with Alan this fueled his craving for fruit. While fruit is certainly a better choice than candy or refined sugar, Alan was eating fifteen to twenty pieces of fruit a day. He thought this was great for his health, but when he had his blood work done, he was actually prediabetic . . . all from eating fresh fruit! This just goes to show you, sugar is sugar. Now that he is off gluten and properly absorbing nutrition, his fruit cravings have subsided and his blood sugar levels are back in check, plus he feels so much better—no bloating, fatigue, or constipation.

To maximize nutrition, digestion, and weight loss, fruit should be eaten on an empty stomach and not combined with any other foods. When we have a substantial release of insulin, we want to make sure that food will be burned off rather than stored as fat. If we have a big breakfast of fruit, eggs, butter, and sausage, the proteins and fats do not cause any rise in blood sugar, but the insulin release spurred by the fruit may lead to the rest of the meal being stored as fat. So if you want Fruit and Protein for breakfast, you would eat your Fruit first, then wait an hour before you have Proteins and Healthy Fats. Again, it will become very clear how to do this when you see the Weekly Menus to come; you'll understand the flow of this process.

Here are the guidelines for eating Fruit:

- Eat Fruit alone, on an empty stomach.

- Eat Fruit alone, one hour before a Protein/Healthy Fats/Vegetable meal.

- For breakfast, eat Fruit alone, then wait at least twenty minutes before Carbohydrates.

- Eat Fruit alone, as a snack at midmorning, or late afternoon.

- As a snack or for dessert, eat Fruit two hours after a meal.

- Fruit is not recommended after dinner, with the occasional exception of berries.

Eat Three Meals a Day

A significant aspect of this program is that we lose weight by eating. Food fuels your metabolism. The shift is that you will be eating nutritious food, rather than the processed, packaged, dead foods found in bags and boxes at the grocery store or in the diet section. For this reason, you can't skip meals. You have to eat. (Isn't that nice?) When you skip meals, you force your body to live off your fat reserves. While this seems like a good idea in the short run, if your body is not receiving nutrition on a steady basis,

Berry Good

The dark, intense color of blueberries, blackberries, and raspberries is a key to the nutrition locked inside; the more intense the color, the higher the antioxidants. Berries are also very high in fiber. By now you are an expert in knowing that fiber reduces the effect of insulin. For this amazing reason, berries get a bit of an exception from the rest of fruits. While you are in the Weight Loss Phase, it's okay, on occasion, to add berries after a meal. This really helps when you are at dinner and everyone is ordering dessert. Get yourself a nice bowl of fresh berries. It's still best if you can wait two hours after your last meal, but this is a place where I teach you how to create only slight imbalances. I would much rather you have a little bit of insulin from berries than completely blow it by ordering a cupcake loaded with sugar and white flour. And I feel great knowing you are building your immune system with all those amazing phytonutrients. Berries can be quite expensive, but at some mass retailers, like Costco, you can find large containers for the same price you might pay for one little container at the grocery store. This allows for fresh berries more often! A luxury, and it's a little easier on the wallet.

it will become trained to store your food as fat, rather than burning it off as fuel. This is the body's natural survival instinct. Low-calorie diets will cause initial weight loss, but then the body will shift into survival mode and hold on to that next meal for fear you will not feed it again soon.

On the Sexy Forever plan, we feed the body at least three times a day, plus snacks as needed. The key is clean, real food, filled with nutrition. This actually increases your metabolism. Plus, once you are giving your body the nutrition it craves, you will require less food to feel satisfied. Some people eat small meals every couple of hours, while others stick to three meals. You have freedom with this program, but you must feed the body, without overeating, in order to get results! You have the opportunity to customize these plans at SexyForever.com/book.

Hydrate

While experts may have varying opinions on many aspects of health, one issue where we generally find consensus is on keeping the body hydrated with water each day. Why is water so important to our bodies? Water assists in all aspects of the functioning of the human body. All living things must have water to survive. People can't live for more than a few days without water. Water is the main ingredient in the fluids of the body's systems. Fluids travel through your body, carrying nutrients and waste to and from all your cells and organs. Water also keeps your joints lubricated.

When your body generates a lot of heat, water comes up through your skin as perspiration, and it evaporates into the air. This process cools down your skin, which cools down your blood, which cools down the whole body. That's why water is especially important when you are exercising or when the weather is hot. Give your body the water it needs! Our bodies lose two to three quarts of water every day and we must replace it. Don't wait until you're thirsty to drink water. If your mouth gets dry and you feel thirsty, you are already experiencing the first sign of dehydration.

Drink eight 8-ounce glasses of water each day. You may need less water if you eat foods that have a lot of water in them, like fruits, vegetables, and soups. Other liquids count toward your water intake. Sodas contain water but are filled with chemicals, sugar, and empty calories, so they are not part of the Sexy Forever plan. Chemicals are not sexy. And sugar causes weight gain . . . definitely not sexy!

Water is also essential in the digestive process. Starting in the mouth, saliva is made mostly of water, and it helps break down food in the mouth. Then your digestive juices are made mostly of gastric acids and water to keep things moving properly. Here's another tip to maximize your digestion; try not to drink too much water with your meals, since it can dilute your digestive juices. Your stomach acids are strongest right before you begin a new meal. These acids break down the food and pass it from the stomach into the intestines. If those acids are diluted, you have less power to process the food. Best to drink your water between meals, or eat at least half of your meal before you drink water to optimize those essential gastric acids.

As for flavored waters, as long as they are free of sugar, artificial sweeteners, or juice, you may have them. Still, my preference is purified, non-carbonated water, maybe with a little lemon. And remember, stay hydrated!

Wait Two Hours Between Meals or Snacks

Remember, when you eat Carbohydrates you will have a rise in your insulin—therefore, I recommend that you don't eat fat, or eat only minimal fats, when you choose to add that Carbohydrate as a snack or to a meal. As a rule, if you are eating a Carbohydrate as a snack, wait two hours before your next Protein/Healthy Fats meal. This will continue to isolate the insulin produced by the carbohydrates. After two hours, you may choose to have a Protein/Healthy Fats meal. The insulin will now be processed and you do not have to worry about the insulin carrying those higher-calorie proteins and fats to the fat reserves. Again, it's important that you do not add even approved Carbohydrates to a meal high in fat.

SUPERFOODS AND SPICES

Superfoods are foods readily available with more natural power than a packed medicine cabinet! These foods are nature's way to reduce your risk of cancer and heart disease, lower your cholesterol, and boost your immune system across the board. Like superheroes, they each have different powers, but all fight for good against evil. Some have a high phytonutrient content, some are excellent sources for essential omega-3s, others are packed with protein or loaded with antioxidants, some are natural digestive cleansers, and more. And they can all be found in their whole, unprocessed state at the local grocery store. These foods are some of the best choices to boost your immune system and give your body the essentials for good health. And they taste delicious! Make it a habit to include them often in your daily meals.

Salmon. This cold-water fish is loaded with omega-3 fatty acids. This good source of monounsaturated fats helps lower cholesterol and the risk of heart disease, plus helps with memory loss, Alzheimer's, and arthritis. Remember to avoid farmed salmon—insist on wild-caught.

Eggs. An excellent source of protein. Look for organic omega-3 and DHA-fortified eggs for added benefits. For those who have a hard time affording organic protein, organic eggs are the least expensive form of organic protein and are versatile for breakfast, lunch, and dinner.

Nuts. They are one of nature's perfect foods, rich in protein, healthy fats, and good carbohydrates. You'll find they are rich in omega-3s, manganese, copper, and ellagic acid (shown to support the immune system and provide anticancer benefits). Nuts are heart-healthy, promote cognitive (brain) function, and provide anti-inflammatory benefits. Even though they contain protein, fat, and carbohydrate, I have categorized them as Carbohydrates in the program, and recommend about ten nuts per serving.

Quinoa. This ancient "grain" from the Incas has a crunchy, nutty flavor. While it may look, taste, and act like a grain, it's actually a relative of leafy greens, like spinach and Swiss chard. This is an excellent choice for vegetarians, because it contains the nutrients of a complete protein, meaning it has all eight essential amino acids! It's also a good source of lysine, which the body uses for tissue growth and repair (and can help heal cold sores, by the way). It's packed with manganese, magnesium, iron, copper, and phosphorus, and studies show it could be beneficial for fighting migraines, diabetes, and atherosclerosis. What I love is that it cooks in minutes and it has a low glycemic index, 35. Therefore we categorize it as a Carbohydrate for this program. Try it warm for breakfast with nonfat milk.

Sweet Potato. If you think sweet potatoes, topped with brown sugar and marshmallows, are just for Thanksgiving, you are sorely mistaken! This amazing vegetable contains root storage proteins with significant antioxidant benefits, including glutathione, which, as we've discussed, is one of nature's most important antioxidants. They are also loaded with beta-carotene, vitamins A and C, manganese, copper, fiber, vitamin

B_6, potassium, and iron. Because they are a little high on the glycemic index (54)—technically they are Insulin Triggers—we will wait until we are on Level 2—Lifestyle Phase to incorporate them, when your cells are cleaned out and ready to absorb their nutritious goodness!

Olive Oil. You know by now what a fan I am of olive oil. This monounsaturated fat has excellent health benefits. In this country, high fat intake usually refers to fake fats in processed foods, including dangerous trans fats. In other parts of the world, high fat intake is actually synonymous with excellent health, because these people eat the right kind of fat! The Mediterranean diet, rich in olive oil, creates a lower incidence of heart disease, diabetes, colon cancer, asthma, and atherosclerosis. A clinical study showed that after six years, those most closely following a Mediterranean diet, rich in olive oil, had half the risk of overall mortality. I buy extra virgin olive oil by the case (much less expensive this way) and I reach for it several times a day.

Tomatoes. By now most of you have heard about the amazing studies on the benefits of lycopene, a phytonutrient. Lycopene is a carotenoid found in tomatoes, and, in fact, is found in higher concentration in cooked tomato products, like tomato sauce and even ketchup (naturally sweetened, please!). This phytonutrient has been proven to have antioxidant and cancer-preventing properties because of its ability to help protect cells and other structures in the body from oxygen damage. Studies have shown lycopene aids in prevention against the following types of cancers: colorectal, prostate, breast, endometrial, lung, and pancreatic. Plus, lycopene has been shown to be a powerful antioxidant in preventing heart disease. I grow my own organic tomatoes, and they are truly nature's gift.

Cruciferous Vegetables: Kale, Broccoli, Red Cabbage

Kale. This dark green leafy vegetable is the undisputed king of the nutrient-dense world of nature. Kale includes ten to fifteen glucosinolates to fight cancer, which work by activating detoxifying enzymes in the liver that help neutralize carcinogenic substances. Just one cup has 88 percent of your vitamin C requirements for the day, plus nearly double the amount of vitamin A you need daily to keep vision and lung health at optimum, in addition to manganese, fiber, calcium, and a host of other nutrients. I love it sautéed with olive oil. So good. So good for you.

Broccoli. While not quite as nutrient dense as kale, broccoli has the same amazing benefits for cancer fighting and cell cleansing. It's an all-around good guy and a staple several times a week in my meals. It's high in vitamins C, K, and A, as well as folate, dietary fiber, manganese, potassium, and more. I love it with olive oil and lemon.

Red Cabbage. Cabbage is packed with anticarcinogenic sulforaphane. Like others in the cruciferous vegetable family, this cancer warrior has been shown to prevent colon cancer, promote proper estrogen metabolism in women, and lower the risk of heart disease. Consumption of cruciferous vegetables is known to reduce the risk of lung, colon, breast, ovarian, and bladder cancer. Now, research reveals that cruciferous vegetables provide significant cardiovascular benefits as well. Green cabbage is good too, but red cabbage provides ten times the nutrients.

Berries. I have already told you about my fondness for berries. Talk about buzzwords in the world of phytonutrients—berries rank the highest in phytonutrients of all fruits, plus they are high in vitamin C and potassium. What does that mean for you? Just by enjoying nature's sweet treats, you can lower your risk of heart disease and cancer. Plus, since we know inflammation is the root of chronic disease, why wouldn't you indulge in berries and benefit from their anti-inflammatory qualities? Go for the deepest-colored berries, such as acai, blueberries, and pomegranates, for the highest antioxidant levels. And be sure to check out Sexy Forever Maqui Juice Blend. I drink one ounce every day.

Yogurt. Loaded with calcium, iodine, riboflavin, and vitamin B_2, this treat helps protect bone health. Studies show yogurt provides excellent bone protection, especially for growing young girls. Yogurt is also revered for its live bacteria cultures (probiotics), proven to help you live longer and fortify the immune system. Added benefits include prevention of yeast infections in women and improvement in cholesterol levels (lowering your bad and raising good). Try the Greek varieties with a little agave nectar—oh my.

Dark Chocolate. I didn't make this one up—dark chocolate is an excellent source of antioxidants. The darker the better; I recommend at least 60 percent cocoa. Those antioxidants found in this delectable treat have been proven to help lower blood pressure. Look for varieties with pure ingredients and low sugar content. If you are eating cheap chocolate, it's all fillers and you're not getting the antioxidant benefits. As with berries, if you are going to stray a little from the strict guidelines, cheat with dark chocolate. It's not part of the program to include chocolate on Detox or Level 1, but it's the best "cheat" if you are going to go there. And it's a staple once you are on Level 2. Have one or two squares in the afternoon, or if everyone else is having dessert, pull out a little stash from your purse to keep you away from the really bad choices.

Spice for Life: Super Herbs and Spices. More of the brilliance of nature—herbs and spices not only provide natural flavorings to enhance and make our food more delicious, they are also an incredible source of antioxidants. Brilliant! You will see in the recipe section that I deliberately add things like turmeric on your eggs and chicken, fresh herbs on seafood and salads, marinades with ginger, and cinnamon sprinkled on yogurt. Yes, these are added for flavor, but they continually act to detoxify the body as well. These antioxidants destroy free radicals and protect your body on a cellular level. So the more herbs and spices you take in, the greater your ability to fight off disease and detoxify your system. Include these herbs and spices liberally in your meals!

Basil	Cayenne pepper
Black pepper	Crushed red pepper flakes

Cumin	Oregano
Curry powder	Paprika
Dill	Rosemary
Fennel	Sage
Garlic (fresh)	Sea salt
Lemon	Tarragon
Lime	Thyme
Mint (fresh)	Turmeric
Nutmeg	Vanilla
Onion	

Coffee. Maybe I've talked myself into this because I really don't want to live in a world without my morning cup of coffee. That being said, I have updated my position on coffee. Simply, caffeine creates an insulin response, so I have always recommended decaf. Like all things, however, I have to adapt my information as I receive it.

To me, it's simply not morning without my coffee, so I've found a way to enjoy a real cup of caffeinated coffee without upsetting my meals. First thing in the morning, I have one cup of real, organic coffee, then I wait an hour before I have my breakfast. This works for me to isolate the insulin response from the caffeine. Oh, and how I love that little perk from the coffee! I have my coffee and usually work out, then have my breakfast.

You can continue to enjoy decaf coffee, but I only recommend Swiss Water process. Chemicals including methylene chloride, ethyl acetate, and formaldehyde are generally used for decaffeination. Users of chemicals typically refer to the decaffeinated coffee as "naturally decaffeinated," which only means that "natural" chemicals are used. Only one company uses pure water and no chemicals in its patented Swiss Water process to extract 99.9 percent of the caffeine. These decaf beans are more healthful and have no chemical residues.

Whether you are interested in regular or Swiss Water process decaf, I have found a company that uses a new, all-natural technique of roasting unadulterated coffee that seals in essential minerals, vitamins, antioxidants, and more normally lost during the roasting process. And the best part about this coffee is that it doesn't upset your stomach! So many of us love our coffee, but can't drink it because of the acid content. Now you can enjoy delicious coffee without bitterness of aftertaste, with those amazing antioxidants (4 to 22 percent of your RDA!) and low acid for the millions with reflux or heartburn. Visit my website for more information.

Now that you have the basic overview of the program, let me take you through the three phases of the plan so you can see what a typical day might look like. Remember, Sexy Forever is a lifestyle plan. Your meals may vary greatly from mine, but this section will give you an idea of how you will enjoy these fabulous foods while the pounds melt away. (For a vast supply of meal plans, join SexyForever.com/book.)

DETOX PHASE: DAYS 1 TO 30

Regardless of how cleanly we have tried to live our lives, we all have stored toxins from the many areas I have discussed at length in the first section of the book. For this reason, the first phase of the Sexy Forever eating plan is the Detox Phase, to clean out your system. During these first thirty days, it's important that you follow the guidelines strictly, but the food has incredible flavor, and I promise you will be full! No deprivation; that only leads to cheating and failure. You will have great food, you won't be hungry, and the best news is that you'll see results quickly as you release the stored sugar and toxins from your cells.

Here is an example of how you will eat during these first thirty days.

Breakfast
Break the fast; while you have been sleeping, your body has gone without food for several hours. Now it's time to eat! Your mother was right, breakfast is the most important meal of the day to charge your metabolism. You have several options for your day's first meal.

Breakfast 1—Fruit meal

Breakfast 2—Carbohydrate meal

Breakfast 3—Fruit, wait twenty minutes, then Carbohydrate meal

Breakfast 4—Protein/HealthyFat/Vegetable meal

Breakfast 1: Fruit Meal

Select any of the fruits from the approved list in the Food Reference Guide. Fruit salad, a fruit smoothie, half a melon—anything that sounds good to you. You just need to avoid bananas, since they are high in starch and are Insulin Triggers. Do not eat anything else with your fruit. If you are having a fruit smoothie, no yogurt, sherbet, or ice cream, just blend fruit (fresh or frozen), a little fruit juice, and ice if you want it slushy. Here are a few examples.

Fruit Meals

- Fruit smoothie made with mangoes, raspberries, and guava juice

- Fruit salad with grapes, melon, and oranges

- An apple

- A bowl of cherries

- Two slices of watermelon

To drink: decaf black coffee or tea, with all-natural sweetener, if desired.

Breakfast 2: Carbohydrate Meal

During the Detox Phase, you are allowed three servings of Carbohydrates (again from the list in the Food Reference Guide). If you choose to eat your Carbohydrates at breakfast, you may have all of them at this time. At breakfast you may combine your Carbohydrates with nonfat dairy products (which are also Carbohydrates) or Vegetables. There are a number of great options for whole-grain carbohydrates, but finding ones that comply with the plan means reading some labels carefully. Just because a product lists "whole grain" on the label doesn't mean it's made with 100 percent whole grains. You must read the whole label and find breads and cereals made with 100 percent whole grains or whole-grain flours. If you see "wheat flour" it's made with white flour. It must be listed as "whole wheat flour" to be a whole grain. Also, make sure there are no added fats, sugars, or fruits. You don't need to worry about the carbohydrates listed on the nutritional panel; you just need to focus on the ingredient list. If all the ingredients are things you see on the Carbohydrate or Vegetable list, then you may include that product. Here are some good choices.

Carbohydrate Meals

- 1 slice whole-wheat toast with ½ cup nonfat cottage cheese (2 servings)

- 1 slice whole-grain toast with sliced tomato and basil (1 serving)

- 1 slice whole-wheat toast with 2 tablespoons peanut butter (3 servings)

- ½ cup nonfat yogurt with 1 cup whole-grain cereal (3 servings)

- ½ cup whole-grain cereal with ½ cup nonfat milk (2 servings)

- 1 cup oatmeal with a splash of nonfat milk and all-natural sweetener (2 servings)

- 1 cup cooked quinoa with a splash of nonfat milk and all-natural sweetener (2 servings)

To drink: decaf coffee or tea, with a little nonfat milk and all-natural sweetener, if desired.

Breakfast 3: Fruit, Wait Twenty Minutes, Then Carbohydrates
Variety! That's what I love about this program. In this option, you enjoy a serving of Fruit, give your body twenty minutes to get the digestion going, and then have one or more servings of Carbohydrates. This breakfast gives you a lot of nutrition from the fresh fruit, then great fiber from the whole-grain carbohydrates. Eating your Fruit, then Carbohydrates in

the morning means the rest of your day will be predominantly made up of Protein, Healthy Fats, and Vegetables. Since fruit and carbs provide you with a lot of energy, the morning is a good time to eat them so you have time to burn off the energy they provide. Alan makes great fruit smoothies, so we usually have a smoothie, then I'll do a little yoga or maybe have my bath, then we enjoy some toast or cereal.

Fruit, Then Carbohydrate Meals

- Fruit smoothie, wait twenty minutes, then 1 slice whole-grain toast with ½ cup nonfat cottage cheese and a sprinkle of cinnamon (2 servings Carbohydrates)

- Fruit salad, wait twenty minutes, then 1 cup oatmeal with a splash of nonfat milk and all-natural sweetener (2 servings Carbohydrates)

- Two tangerines, wait twenty minutes, then 1 cup puffed wheat cereal with ½ cup nonfat milk (3 servings Carbohydrates)

- An apple, wait twenty minutes, then ½ cup whole-grain cereal flakes with ½ cup nonfat milk (2 servings Carbohydrates)

To drink: decaf coffee or tea (drink black with fruit or add nonfat milk with Carbohydrates, plus an all-natural sweetener, if desired).

Breakfast 4: Protein, Healthy Fats, and Vegetables Meal
If you enjoy the traditional bacon-and-eggs type of breakfast, this is an excellent choice. Again, you have so much variety here from which to choose. Eggs can be boiled, scrambled, fried, or poached, using butter or olive oil, and served with vegetables. This makes for a very satisfying breakfast. As always, if you can afford organic eggs, this is your best choice. Sauté some fresh vegetables in olive oil, like mushrooms and spinach, and add beaten eggs for an omelette or a scramble. You can even top them with a sprinkle of cheese or a dollop of sour cream. You can create all sorts of combinations, as long as you work from the approved lists in the book.

Protein, Healthy Fats, and Vegetable Meals

- Eggs fried in butter, served with turkey bacon and sliced tomatoes

- Scrambled eggs with sautéed spinach, mushrooms, and grated Swiss cheese

- Omelette with sautéed asparagus, cheddar cheese, and sausage

- Poached eggs and Canadian bacon, with sautéed spinach and hollandaise sauce

- Soft-boiled eggs with a side of sausage and sautéed zucchini

To drink: decaf coffee or tea with cream and all-natural sweetener, if desired.

Lunch and Dinner

For lunch and dinner you will be starting with Protein, then adding Healthy Fats and Vegetables. This means you may choose salads with fresh vegetables, sliced meats, and full-fat dressing; soups with poultry and vegetables; seafood entrees with butter sauces and fresh vegetables; marinated and grilled steak with salads and vegetables; and roasted chicken with pan drippings and sautéed greens.

You have so much to choose from, and the best news is that these meals are loaded with flavor. You just want to make sure none of your proteins are dusted or coated with flour and that you do not add or consume any flour or thickeners in your sauces. These hidden starches are Insulin Triggers and can send this meal to the fat reserves. It's okay to have Healthy Fats with these meals. And make sure these meals are balanced with plenty of Vegetables. Eating this way gives you all those essential nutrients and natural fiber.

Protein, Healthy Fats, and Vegetable Meals

- Caesar salad with grilled chicken or shrimp (no croutons)

- Cobb salad with chicken, bacon, egg, tomato, blue cheese, green onions, and full-fat salad dressing (without Insulin Triggers)

- Taco salad with romaine lettuce, seasoned ground beef, cheddar cheese, sour cream, and salsa (no beans, no chips)

- Egg salad made with celery and mayo, served in butter lettuce cups with green onions

- Chopped Italian salad with salami, mozzarella, pepperoncini, onions, and Italian dressing

- Roasted chicken with pan drippings, steamed broccoli with olive oil and lemon, sautéed kale

- Grilled steak, green salad and Italian dressing plus cherry tomatoes, steamed asparagus

- Cheeseburger, protein style (no bun—serve in a crunchy lettuce cup), with sugar-free ketchup and mayo, sliced tomato and onion, side salad

- Grilled lamb chops with garlic and rosemary, green beans, sautéed Swiss chard

- Sautéed pork chops with thyme, lemon, and olive oil, steamed cauliflower and broccoli

- Pan-fried salmon and lemon-butter sauce, sautéed snap peas

To drink: water, mineral water, decaf coffee or tea with cream and all-natural sweetener, if desired.

Putting It All Together

Now that you see the options for breakfast, lunch, and dinner, let me show you how you might put it all together for a week's worth of meals and snacks. Remember, this is just for the Detox Phase. You will have a little more freedom when we move to Level 1. In Detox, we want to really unload those stored toxins and allow your body to release the stored sugar and fat from your cells.

THE DEAL WITH DAIRY

Dairy contains varying levels of carbohydrates, depending upon how much milk is left in the end product. For example, non-fat milk has carbohydrates and no fat. Cream and cheeses (hard or semi-soft) have fat, but virtually no carbohydrates. Whole milk, low-fat milk, wet cheeses (cottage cheese, ricotta cheese, fresh mozzarella), and yogurt are in between—with some carbohydrates and some fat. So how do we categorize them for Sexy Forever?

Healthy Fats *Enjoy these foods according to guidelines for Healthy Fats.*
Butter
Cream
Cheese (hard or semi-soft)
Cream cheese (full fat)
Sour cream (full fat)

Carbohydrates *Count each serving toward your Carbohydrate count.*
Nonfat cottage cheese
Nonfat milk
Nonfat yogurt
Nonfat ricotta cheese

Healthy Fats with Carbohydrates *You may enjoy these products with Healthy Fats as long as you also count each serving toward your Carbohydrate count.*
Low-fat or whole milk
Cottage cheese
Ricotta cheese
Fresh mozzarella
Yogurt

Avoid

Some nonfat or low-fat dairy products contain added starch or thickeners to make up for the missing fat (especially sour cream and cream
cheese). Check ingredients lists for modified food starch, gums, or thickening agents. Better to avoid these products and use full-fat products in
a Protein/Healthy Fats meal.

DETOX PHASE: ONE WEEK'S WORTH OF MEAL PLANS

Sunday

8:00   Coffee, black*

9:00   Breakfast—Protein, Healthy Fats, Vegetables meal
       Scrambled eggs with spinach, feta cheese, and tomatoes
       Side of turkey sausage

11:00 Snack—Fruit
       1 apple

12:30 Lunch—Protein, Healthy Fats, Vegetables meal
       Baby green lettuce salad with chicken, sun-dried tomatoes,
       goat cheese, and balsamic vinaigrette

3:30   Snack—Carbohydrates and Vegetables
       2 brown rice cakes with tomato salsa

6:00   Dinner—Protein, Healthy Fats, Vegetables meal
       Salad with cherry tomatoes and cucumbers, plus blue cheese
       dressing
       Pan-fried Dover sole with lemon-butter sauce
       Steamed broccoli with Parmesan cheese

Monday

6:00   Coffee, black*

7:00   Breakfast—Fruit, wait 20 minutes, then Carbohydrates

* *You may add an all-natural sweetener, like SomerSweet, if desired.*

Fruit smoothie (frozen peaches, raspberries, orange juice)

20-minute wait

1 slice whole-grain toast with ½ cup nonfat cottage cheese, sprinkled with cinnamon

10:00   Snack—Healthy Fats

Slice of cheddar cheese

12:30   Lunch—Protein, Healthy Fats, Vegetables meal

Caesar salad with grilled shrimp (no croutons)

3:30   Snack—Fruit

1 mango

7:00   Dinner—Protein, Healthy Fats, Vegetables meal

Roasted chicken with olive oil, lemon, and thyme

Broccoli Limone—steamed, then tossed with garlic, olive oil, and lemon juice

Salad with butter lettuce, fennel, purple cabbage, olive oil, and lemon

9:00   Snack—Healthy Fats

Slice of Jarlsberg cheese

Tuesday

7:00   Coffee, black*

8:00   Breakfast—Protein, Healthy Fats, Vegetables meal

Eggs fried in butter

Crisp bacon

Sliced tomatoes

10:00   Snack—Fruit

A bowl of cherries

10:30   Snack—Carbohydrates

10 almonds

12:30   Lunch—Protein, Healthy Fats, Vegetables meal

Bowl of chicken and vegetable soup (no pasta or rice)

Wedge of iceberg with blue cheese dressing and cherry tomatoes

* *You may add an all-natural sweetener, like SomerSweet, if desired.*

2:30   Snack—Fruit
½ cantaloupe

3:30   Snack—Carbohydrates
1 brown rice cake

6:30   Dinner—Protein, Healthy Fats, Vegetables meal
Salad with white wine vinaigrette
Pork chops with fried sage leaves
Green beans sautéed in butter
Slice of cheesecake made with cream cheese, sour cream, eggs, and all-natural sweetener (no sugar)

Wednesday

6:00   Coffee, black*

7:00   Breakfast—Fruit, wait 20 minutes, then Carbohydrates
Casaba melon
20-minute wait
½ toasted whole-wheat bagel, 1 cup nonfat Greek yogurt with agave nectar

11:00   Snack—Protein
1 hard-boiled egg

1:00   Lunch—Protein, Healthy Fats, Vegetables meal
Taco salad with romaine lettuce, meat, salsa, sour cream, cheddar cheese (no beans, rice, or chips)

4:00   Snack—Fruit
1 bunch grapes

7:00   Dinner—Protein, Healthy Fats, Vegetables meal
Chicken piccata (no flour)
Radicchio and arugula salad with shaved Parmesan, olive oil, and lemon
Sautéed zucchini in olive oil
SUZANNE Raspberry Mousse made with heavy cream

* *You may add an all-natural sweetener, like SomerSweet, if desired.*

Thursday

6:30   Coffee, black*

7:30   Breakfast—Fruit
       Fruit smoothie with frozen mango, peaches, strawberries, and
       passionfruit juice

9:30   Snack—Carbohydrates
       1 slice whole-grain toast with 2 tablespoons peanut butter

12:30 Lunch—Protein, Healthy Fats, Vegetables meal
       Rotisserie chicken
       Caesar salad (no croutons)
       Celery sticks with ranch dressing

3:00   Snack—Fruit
       Bowl of fresh pineapple

7:00   Dinner—Protein, Healthy Fats, Vegetables meal
       Beef Bourguignon—beef, onions, tomatoes, celery, wine, herbs
       Mashed celery root with butter and sour cream
       Caramelized fennel with olive oil and butter

Friday

6:00   Coffee, black*

7:00   Breakfast—Fruit, wait 20 minutes, then Carbohydrates
       Bowl of fresh berries
       20-minute wait
       1 cup Uncle Sam's cereal with ½ cup nonfat milk

12:00 Lunch—Protein, Healthy Fats, Vegetables meal
       Chicken stir-fry with snap peas, green beans, broccoli, onion,
       soy sauce, olive oil

3:00   Snack—Protein
       Hard-boiled egg

5:00   Snack—Fruit
       1 apple

7:30   Dinner—Protein, Healthy Fats, Vegetables meal

* *You may add an all-natural sweetener, like SomerSweet, if desired.*

Turkey chili with cheddar cheese and sour cream

Coleslaw salad with green and purple cabbage, red onion, and red wine vinaigrette

Saturday

7:00   Coffee, black*

8:00   Breakfast—Protein, Healthy Fats, Vegetables meal

Zucchini frittata with eggs, olive oil, zucchini, Parmesan, fresh basil

Side of breakfast sausage

10:30 Snack—Carbohydrates and Vegetables

Celery sticks with 2 tablespoons peanut butter

1:00   Lunch—Protein, Healthy Fats, Vegetables meal

Sliced turkey and Swiss cheese roll-ups

Raw red bell peppers, snap peas, and green beans with dip

3:30   Snack—Fruit

Bowl of fresh berries

7:00   Dinner—Protein, Healthy Fats, Vegetables meal

Steak fajitas with sautéed peppers and onions (no tortillas)

Steamed broccoli

Salad with jicama, cherry tomatoes, and cilantro lime dressing

Now you can see how the flow of your days might pan out, so to speak. Your meals do not have to look like mine, but you will see how we get all the food groups in each day, to nurture our bodies with everything they need to thrive. And you can see there is plenty of food! When you are hungry, there is always something you can eat. You will even see how I have added some desserts in there, as long as they are made with only Proteins, Healthy Fats, and low-glycemic-index natural sweeteners. You may enjoy them in moderation, even in the Detox Phase. (For detailed meal plans, more recipes, and daily guidance from me, check out my on-line program at SexyForever.com/book. It makes it so easy!)

---

* *You may add an all-natural sweetener, like SomerSweet, if desired.*

LEVEL 1—WEIGHT LOSS PHASE (DAY 31 UNTIL YOU HIT YOUR GOAL WEIGHT)

After the first thirty days you enter the Weight Loss Phase, where you will remain until you achieve your goal weight. I understand how vitally important it is that this phase is a lifestyle you can live with. If it's too restrictive, you may feel too deprived and bail out. I don't want you to revert to your old eating habits! As we transition to Level 1, the guidelines are still clear, but I allow you some moderation in order to make the plan livable. Your health and well-being are too important; compliance to the program is vital for success. That's why I have made sure you have plenty of delicious food and snacks to keep you on track. And you even have access to desserts!

In this phase, we use the basis of the Detox Phase, and we add a little bit more freedom. Instead of three servings of Carbohydrates per day, you can choose up to four servings each day (although you don't *have* to eat all four). Plus, you have the choice to add Carbohydrates to a Protein, Healthy Fats, and Vegetables meal. If you decide to add carbohydrates to that protein meal, do not add more than one serving at each meal. And when you add a serving of Carbohydrates to a Protein meal, watch out for the amount of fats. I'm not going to give you a quantity, but if you follow the guidelines, your common sense will tell you what is appropriate.

When you add that whole-grain Carbohydrate, you'll release a small amount of insulin as a result of the meal. So if you'd like a piece of sugarless cheesecake at the end of a meal, don't include that Carbohydrate! Or if you want a couple of slices of Brie before a dinner of roasted chicken with pan drippings, skip adding the ½ cup of wild rice. I would choose to add that serving of approved Carbohydrate if I were having, say, a grilled chicken breast with olive oil, steamed broccoli, and a green salad with a vinaigrette. With that meal, it would be perfectly balanced to add a ½ cup of brown rice because the meal is not overloaded with fats. Remember, there is virtually no insulin response from the Protein, Healthy Fats, and Vegetables meal, so those foods will not be stored as fat—that's why you can have pork carnitas with sour cream and salsa. (How much do you love me? So much . . . I know.) But remember, when you choose a meal higher in fats, don't add the Carbohydrate.

Have even more fun in Level 1 with chocolate! Dark chocolate, with a cocoa content of at least 60 percent, includes wonderful antioxidants from the cacao bean and is generally low in sugar. I've found that once your weight loss is in full swing, most people can include one or two squares of high-quality chocolate as a treat. I might have this little treat a couple of times a week. The best time of the day to enjoy it is as a snack in the afternoon. Eat your chocolate alone, not with other foods. Again, you will have a bit of an insulin response because of the sugar and carbohydrates, so only have one or two squares, and only once (okay, maybe twice a week, if you are losing steadily). Once you get to Level 2, you will see that high-quality dark chocolate will be your dessert of choice!

If at any time in Level 1 you feel your weight loss is stalling, return to the Detox guidelines to get things moving again. When you come back to the Weight Loss Phase, perhaps pull back a bit on the additions to ensure your weight loss remains steady. Again, you customize the plan to suit your needs. If you are doing better eating fewer Carbohydrates, then do not add more to your meals in Level 1.

LEVEL 1—WEIGHT LOSS PHASE:
A WEEK'S WORTH OF MENUS FOR DELICIOUS WEIGHT LOSS

Sunday
7:00   Coffee, black*
8:00   Breakfast—Protein, Healthy Fats, Vegetables meal
        Huevos rancheros with fried eggs, sautéed onions, salsa, cheese, and sour cream (no tortillas, beans, or guacamole)
10:30   Snack—Fruit
        1 peach

* *You may add an all-natural sweetener, like SomerSweet, if desired.*

1:00   Lunch—Protein, Healthy Fats, Vegetables meal with
1 Carbohydrate
Sliced turkey, romaine lettuce, sliced tomato, red onion, and
mustard on 1 slice whole-wheat bread

3:00   Snack—Fruit
Papaya cubes

7:00   Dinner—Protein, Healthy Fats, Vegetables meal with
1 Carbohydrate
Pan-roasted salmon with olive oil, soy sauce, agave, and green
onions
Sautéed snow peas and water chestnuts
½ cup brown rice

Monday

6:00   Coffee, black*

7:00   Breakfast—Fruit, wait 20 minutes, then Carbohydrates
Fruit smoothie with frozen pineapple, strawberries,
blueberries, and peach juice
20-minute wait
1 cup Irish oats with a splash of nonfat milk*

10:30   Snack—Protein
1 slice cheese

1:00   Lunch—Protein, Healthy Fats, Vegetables meal
Caesar salad with grilled chicken (no croutons)
Side of broccoli

4:00   Snack—Carbohydrate
1 brown rice cake

7:00   Dinner—Protein, Healthy Fats, Vegetables meal with
1 Carbohydrate
Sautéed shrimp with grapeseed oil, lemon, garlic, ginger,
green beans, and snap peas
½ cup brown rice

* *You may add an all-natural sweetener, like SomerSweet, if desired.*

Tuesday

6:30   Coffee, black*

7:30   Breakfast—Protein, Healthy Fats with 1 Carbohydrate
       SUZANNE Protein Shake blended with 6 ounces water,
       2 ounces heavy cream, ice

11:00   Snack—Carbohydrates, Vegetables
       Celery sticks with 1 tablespoon peanut or almond butter

1:00   Lunch—Protein, Healthy Fats, Vegetables meal with
       1 Carbohydrate
       Spinach salad with grilled chicken, goat cheese, sun-dried
       tomatoes, balsamic vinaigrette, and a handful of toasted
       pine nuts

4:00   Snack—Fruit
       2 oranges

7:30   Dinner—Protein, Healthy Fats, Vegetables meal
       Crab legs with melted butter and lemon
       Steamed broccoli
       Green salad with olive oil and lemon
       SUZANNE Crème Brûlée

Wednesday

6:00   Coffee, black*

7:00   Breakfast—Fruit, wait 20 minutes, then Carbohydrates
       Bowl of fresh berries
       20-minute wait
       1 cup Uncle Sam's cereal with ½ cup nonfat milk

10:00   Snack—Protein
       String cheese

1:00   Lunch—Protein, Healthy Fats, Vegetables meal, plus
       1 Carbohydrate
       Grilled chicken breast with lime and olive oil, and pico de
       gallo (fresh tomato salsa)

* *You may add an all-natural sweetener, like SomerSweet, if desired.*

Raw jicama sticks
½ cup black beans

4:30 Snack—Fruit
1 nectarine

7:30 Dinner—Protein, Healthy Fats, Vegetables meal
Turkey meat loaf with marinara sauce
Steamed asparagus

Thursday

6:30 Coffee, black*

7:30 Breakfast—Protein, Healthy Fats, Vegetables meal with
1 Carbohydrate
Scrambled eggs with asparagus, olive oil, and basil
1 slice whole-grain toast with olive oil

10:00 Snack—Fruit
2 slices honeydew melon

12:00 Lunch—Protein, Healthy Fats, Vegetables meal with
1 Carbohydrate
Chopped Italian salad with turkey, mozzarella, roasted red
pepper, garbanzo beans, and Italian dressing

3:00 Snack—Fruit
1 pear

6:00 Dinner—Protein, Healthy Fats, Vegetables meal with
1 Carbohydrate
Thai red curry chicken with green beans
½ cup brown jasmine rice

Friday

6:00 Coffee, black*

7:00 Breakfast—Carbohydrates
1 slice whole-grain toast with 1 tablespoon peanut butter

10:00 Snack—Fruit
2 plums

* *You may add an all-natural sweetener, like SomerSweet, if desired.*

12:30   Lunch—Protein, Healthy Fats, Vegetables meal with
         1 Carbohydrate
         Mongolian BBQ stir-fry with beef, green onions, broccoli,
         cabbage, onions, mushrooms, olive oil, garlic, red chili
         pepper, and soy sauce
         ½ cup brown rice

4:00   Snack—Fruit
         1 mango

7:00   Dinner—Protein, Healthy Fats, Vegetables meal
         Baby lamb chops with rosemary, olive oil, and garlic
         Grilled artichoke with lemon butter
         Green salad with slices of goat cheese, pear tomatoes, and
         champagne vinaigrette
         SUZANNE Chocolate Mousse

Saturday
7:00   Coffee, black*

8:00   Breakfast—Fruit
         Fruit smoothie with strawberries, blackberries, raspberries,
         and orange juice

10:30   Snack—Protein and Carbohydrate
         1 SUZANNE Protein Bar

12:30   Lunch—Protein, Healthy Fats, Vegetables meal with
         1 Carbohydrate
         Chicken broth with chicken, celery, parsnips, and parsley
         1 piece whole-grain baguette

3:30   Snack—Fruit
         2 slices watermelon

7:00   Dinner—Protein, Healthy Fats, Vegetables meal with
         1 Carbohydrate
         Roasted chicken leg and thigh with olive oil and sage leaves
         Sautéed kale with olive oil and butter

* *You may add an all-natural sweetener, like SomerSweet, if desired.*

Steamed broccoli

½ cup wild rice

For customized meal plans, printable shopping lists, recipe index, and daily support, join SexyForever.com/book.

LEVEL 2—LIFESTYLE PHASE

I am often asked, "Suzanne, how will I know when to move to Level 2?" I say it's less of a move and more like a transition. The basic guidelines of the Sexy Forever plan will remain a part of your lifestyle, well, forever. You will continue to fill your meals with excellent choices of Protein with Healthy Fats and Vegetables. You will continue to eat whole-grain Carbohydrates as a rule, but now you might add some of those high-starch vegetables (like sweet potatoes, potatoes, corn, or carrots) on occasion. You will continue to eat fruit alone as a general rule, but now that your cells are cleaned out, you might enjoy dessert every now and then—perhaps a delicious low-sugar berry cobbler!

You will see that Level 2 is really very similar to Level 1, but with a little more cheating. If you think you can go back to eating processed food, fast food, and fake food, you will quickly watch all of your success slip through your fingers and you will gain back the weight you lost. Don't let this happen to you! This is not a diet; it's a way of eating that will keep you healthy and fit forever.

Now that you have achieved your goal weight, it's not a license to stuff your face with churros, burritos made with white-flour tortillas, fried fish and chips, cakes, cookies, and pies. As you know, it takes much longer to lose the weight than it does to put it back on!

Here is the shift you need to make in your thinking. You have reached your goal weight. The body you now have is your ideal weight. This weight should not be the exception in the cycle of your life. It will be the rule. The roller coaster is over. The ride has stopped. Now it's time to live your life. You now have the knowledge and the capacity to be Sexy Forever! This does not mean that you live on a diet forever—who wants that? It does mean you have shifted your thinking and created a new lifestyle. You have achieved this goal because you have learned how to nurture your body with proper nutrition. You have learned how to eat sweets in moderation, with all-natural low-glycemic-index choices that do not throw you off the program.

Now that your cells are cleaned out (which you can verify because you are no longer thick through the middle), you may incorporate Protein, Healthy Fats, Vegetables, and Carbohydrates at each meal. You do not need to count a thing! Think of a traditional balanced meal, like protein with a lovely sauce, a starch, and a vegetable. Now select sensible portions and you have mastered Level 2. It really is not that difficult—it's just a discipline you must adopt for life. Let's take a look at the freedoms we will enjoy as we eat this way.

Adding Carbohydrates to Protein, Healthy Fats, and Vegetables

Adding a serving of Carbohydrates can now become commonplace, as long as balance and moderation are considered. Let's say you are going out for Italian food. You will still pass over options like the meatball sandwich on the white roll, spaghetti with meatballs, or pizza. Instead, you will choose the steak, chicken, or seafood entree served with mixed vegetables, but now it's okay to add the lovely potatoes that might come with it. Remember portions—continue to use the guideline of roughly ½ cup of starch when combining it with Protein and Fats. Have the dinner salad, too, and now you don't have to be so concerned if it might have a touch of sugar in the dressing. If you are making mostly good choices, these small imbalances will not get in your way. Plus, now your world is open to enjoying those high-starch vegetables (carrots, corn, potatoes, sweet potatoes) on occasion. These are categorized as Carbohydrates, so take moderate portions, and use a bit of caution not to overdo it.

This is not a license to have a daily plate of french fries! That would not be a good choice. But you can enjoy the occasional half a baked potato or a small portion of baked sweet potato fries. Of course, a couple of times a year you might enjoy that slice of pizza, plate of pasta, or hot, salty fries! Or perhaps your body can handle that type of imbalance once a month. Just as you customized Level 1 with the quantities of food and choices that worked for you, you will now customize Level 2—Lifestyle Phase with the treats that are most important to you. How do you know if you are making the right choices? Your weight! If you start to see the pounds creep up, don't ignore it! Get on top of it right away and go back to making better choices.

Fruit

For the most part, I still continue to eat my Fruit alone. Once you know the insulin response, you just don't freely add fruit back to your meals. Now that you are at Level 2, the place you can loosen up even more is with the berries. Again, it's that high fiber content. I do not think twice about eating berries with whipped cream after a meal. My system can handle it. Even better, I might have some dark chocolate fondue with strawberries! Yum. I might also have an all-fruit jam on my whole-grain toast or whole-grain pancakes. Yes, there's natural sugar in there, but my system is clean and can handle it. I also will choose berries to top whole-grain tarts or to use as fillings in whole-wheat pastry crust. Or a berry cobbler—these are all good choices for those times when you choose to have dessert. In addition, you have likely come across whole-grain cereals that do not have any added sugar, but they use fruit juice as a sweetener. Again, you might try incorporating these during the Lifestyle Phase if you are bored with the other cereal selections. Just don't overdo it! Keep those clean cells of yours neat and tidy so they continue to burn sugar as fuel!

Sugar and the Slippery Slope

For me, sugar is truly my Achilles' heel. Once I start back on it, it's like an evil demon that sucks me in and starts that addictive mechanism. A nibble becomes an occasional dessert, then a daily occurrence, and before I know it, sugar is back in my diet and I have gained five pounds. I will look at Alan and say, "I don't know what happened—I have put on five pounds!" And my darling husband will say, "You've been eating every dessert in sight!" Ha ha. Watch out for this Evil White Sugar Witch! She will suck you in. Use her angelic counterpart—All-Natural SomerSweet.

That being said, you now have the option to add a little bit of sugar and not worry that your body will immediately store it as fat. This is the benefit of the hard work you have done to clean out those cells. Once you have healed your metabolism and detoxified your system you should be able to handle a bit of an imbalance. Just don't behave like me! Or else Alan will remind you that you are being naughty and you will be punished by putting the pounds back on!

I don't worry about a little bit of sugar in sauces or salad dressings (whereas on Detox and Level 1 you should be vigilant about searching for hidden sugars). I will continue to have low- or no-sugar desserts. Dark chocolate is still your best bet. Chocolate flourless cake, molten chocolate cake, chocolate soufflé, chocolate torte—anything that has predominantly eggs, healthy fats, and chocolate! Other good low-sugar desserts are cheesecake, crème brûlée, mousse, and high-quality ice cream that is not filled with a bunch of candy. But if you are going to eat those desserts high in fats, again, do not add carbohydrates to that meal.

White-Flour Warning

Now that I have adapted to a life without white flour, I have too much information and too many benefits to turn back to white bread and pasta. I still choose whole grains because I actually like the taste of them better. The earthiness of the whole grain is much more appealing than its white counterpart. I also continue to avoid white flour in my sauces because I am so used to having my sauces without it. I find the thick sauces gloppy; I much prefer pan juices. Where I miss that white flour is in cake. I really love cake. I don't eat it very often, but when I decide to blow it on white flour and sugar, it's usually with a slice of birthday cake. I only do it a couple of times a year—and only if I am looking and feeling great. If I am feeling a little thick, I will not go there (though I might just have a finger of frosting—I love it!). Just don't go there too often. Don't blow it! Enjoy your new figure, and indulge every now and then.

Portion Size

Now that you are in great shape, commit to enjoying your life of moderation. Do you know how much we eat in this country compared to other countries? Our portions are obscene! When you go to France you might start with a lovely salad. Then you might have 4 ounces of protein, with a small portion of rice or potato and some wonderful vegetables. Then you might have a selection of cheeses, followed by dessert . . . but it's only a few bites of something rich and wonderful. I guarantee you they are not going to a frozen yogurt shop with 24-ounce servings topped with candy and cookies! Moderation. Portion control. Eat great food in reasonable portions and the world will be your oyster. You know how to do it, because you have done an amazing job getting here! Keep up the good work.

Wine

I also find I can add red wine in moderation on Level 2. I can enjoy a glass or two of wine once or twice a week, and red wine has been shown to have beneficial antioxidants. This does not mean share a bottle of wine each night with your spouse—that's too much! I treat wine like a dessert—I usually will choose either wine or dessert. For example, I would not have a potato with dinner, plus a glass of wine, plus a sugar dessert. All three would be too much for me.

Below you'll find a sample week for the Lifestyle Phase. Your meals will vary greatly from this, but it will give you an idea of how I eat most days of the year. You will see I eat several of my meals with Detox or Level 1 guidelines. This is how to keep the balance. And remember, while I have not listed portion sizes, eat reasonably . . . about 6 ounces of protein, ½ cup carbohydrate, and as many low-starch vegetables as you need to feel full. And enjoy high Insulin Triggers, such as wine, corn, potatoes, or dessert every now and then.

LEVEL 2—LIFESTYLE PHASE:
A WEEK'S WORTH OF MENUS FOR DELICIOUS MEALS

Sunday

7:30   Coffee, black*

8:30   Breakfast—Protein, Healthy Fats, Vegetables, and Carbohydrates

---

* *You may add an all-natural sweetener, like SomerSweet, if desired.*

Omelette with sausage and cheese
1 slice whole-grain toast with butter
12:00   Lunch—Protein, Healthy Fats, Vegetables, and Carbohydrates
Chopped Italian salad with salami, tomatoes, garbanzo
beans, mozzarella cheese, and sesame oil vinaigrette
3:00   Snack—Fruit
Mango
7:30   Dinner—Protein, Healthy Fats, Vegetables, and
Carbohydrates
Shrimp stir-fry with lemon, garlic, ginger, green beans, and
brown rice
Lemon curd tart with whole-wheat crust

Monday
6:30   Coffee, black*
7:30   Breakfast—Fruit, then Carbohydrates
Fruit smoothie with peaches, strawberries, orange juice,
and ice
20-minute wait
Irish steel-cut oats with nonfat milk*
10:30   Snack—Protein
Hard-boiled egg
12:00   Lunch—Protein, Healthy Fats, Vegetables
Chicken Caesar salad—no croutons
3:00   Snack—Fruit, Carbohydrates
2 squares dark chocolate and fresh blueberries
7:30   Dinner—Protein, Healthy Fats, Vegetables, and
Carbohydrates
Pan-fried pork chops with olive oil and thyme, steamed
asparagus, baked sweet potato fries
A glass of red wine

*   *You may add an all-natural sweetener, like SomerSweet, if desired.*

Tuesday

7:30   Coffee, black*

8:30   Breakfast—Fruit

        Half a honeydew melon

10:00 Snack—Carbohydrates

        10 walnuts

12:00 Lunch—Protein, Healthy Fats, Vegetables

        Cobb salad with turkey, cheese, avocado, bacon, tomato, cucumber with blue cheese dressing

3:00   Snack—Protein, Healthy Fats, and Carbohydrates

        SUZANNE Protein Shake—Mocha, made with water, ice, and a splash of cream

7:30   Dinner—Protein, Healthy Fats, Vegetables, Insulin Trigger, then Fruit

        Rib-eye steak, steamed broccoli, half a baked potato with butter and sour cream

        Bowl of fresh blackberries

Wednesday

7:30   Coffee, black*

8:30   Breakfast—Fruit, 20-minute wait, then Carbohydrates

        Fruit smoothie with papaya, pineapple, guava juice, and ice

        20-minute wait

        Bowl of Uncle Sam's cereal and nonfat milk

10:30 Snack—Protein

        String cheese

12:00 Lunch—Protein, Healthy Fats, Vegetables

        Grilled chicken breast

        Chopped Israeli salad with cucumber, peppers, and tomatoes, olive oil, lemon, and sea salt

        Piece of Brie cheese

* *You may add an all-natural sweetener, like SomerSweet, if desired.*

3:00   Snack—Carbohydrates
         10 macadamia nuts

7:00   Dinner—Protein, Healthy Fats, Vegetables
         Green salad with butter lettuce and fennel
         Grilled lamb chops with rosemary and thyme
         Grilled radicchio with olive oil and balsamic vinegar
         SUZANNE Chocolate Mousse, made with heavy cream

Thursday

7:30   Coffee, black*

8:30   Breakfast—Protein, Healthy Fats, Vegetables
         Two eggs fried in olive oil with turmeric, cayenne, and paprika
         Sliced tomatoes with fresh basil and olive oil

10:30   Snack—Carbohydrates
         10 hazelnuts

12:00   Lunch—Protein, Healthy Fats, Vegetables, and Carbohydrates
         Chinese chicken salad with romaine lettuce and cashews, with
         sesame oil and rice wine vinegar dressing

3:00   Snack—Fruit
         Fuji apple slices

7:30   Dinner—Protein, Healthy Fats, Vegetables, and
         Carbohydrates
         Chicken soup with celery, carrots, parsley, and wild rice
         SUZANNE Crème Brûlée

Friday

6:30   Coffee, black*

7:30   Breakfast—Fruit, 20-minute wait, then Carbohydrates
         2 tangerines
         20-minute wait
         Amaranth flakes with nonfat milk

10:30   Snack—Protein
         Slice of cheddar cheese

* *You may add an all-natural sweetener, like SomerSweet, if desired.*

12:00   Lunch—Protein, Healthy Fats, Vegetables
        Cheeseburger in lettuce leaves with tomato, grilled onions,
        and no-sugar ketchup
6:30   Dinner—Protein, Healthy Fats, Vegetables, and Insulin Trigger
        Roasted chicken with pan drippings
        Tuscan smashed potatoes with butter and olive oil
        Sautéed kale with olive oil
        Glass of red wine

Saturday

7:30   Coffee, black*
8:30   Breakfast—Protein, Healthy Fats, Vegetables, and Insulin Triggers
        Huevos Rancheros with corn tortillas, eggs, cheese, and salsa
12:00   Lunch—Protein, Healthy Fats, and Vegetables
        Greek salad with lettuce, tomatoes, feta cheese, olives,
        red onion, cucumber
3:00   Snack—Fruit
        Peach
7:30   Dinner—Protein, Healthy Fats, Vegetables, and Carbohydrates
        Green Chile Verde chicken made in the slow cooker with
        SUZANNE Chile Verde sauce
        Quinoa with crispy fried shallots
        Grilled asparagus with lemon and olive oil

Again, this is just an example of what I might eat on a normal day, in a
normal week. If there was a birthday party, I may have had a few bites of
that birthday cake! But as you can see, you are still living on the program.
If you abandon the nutrition plan, you will also have to abandon your new-
found health and slim body . . . and I know you don't want that. Live a little
(as in only cheat a little), if you want to live a lot! One of the wonderful
aspects of this program is sharing tips with likeminded people. I encourage
you to share your success stories with me at SexyForever.com/book.

* *You may add an all-natural sweetener, like SomerSweet, if desired.*

THE EATING PLAN

YOUR SEXY FOREVER CHEAT SHEET

1. Eliminate Insulin Triggers and Bad Fats.

2. Commit to clean, real, organic food.

3. Choose Protein with Healthy Fats and Vegetables at most meals.

4. Eat the right Carbohydrates—Detox: 3 per day, Level 1—Weight Loss: 4 per day.

5. Eat Fruits alone, on an empty stomach.

6. Eat three meals a day, until satisfied and comfortably full. Add snacks as needed.

7. Drink eight 8-ounce glasses of water each day.

8. Wait two hours between meals or snacks if switching from a Carbohydrate to a Protein/Healthy Fats meal or vice versa.

Protein

Meat	Poultry
Eggs	Seafood

Healthy Fats

Butter	Mayonnaise
Cheese	Olive oil
Cream	Sour cream

Vegetables

Asparagus	Green beans
Broccoli	Lettuce
Cauliflower	Mushrooms
Celery	Spinach
Cucumber	Tomato
Eggplant	Zucchini

Carbohydrates

Beans

Brown rice

Nonfat milk products

100 percent whole-grain
  bread, cereal, or pasta

Wild rice

Fruit

Apples

Berries

Grapes

Mangoes

Melons

Nectarines

Oranges

Papaya

Peaches

Pears

Plums

ELIMINATE INSULIN TRIGGERS

Sugar

Corn syrup

Honey

Maple syrup

Molasses

Sugar

Starches

Bananas

Beets

Carrots

Corn

Pasta made from semolina or
  white flour

Popcorn

Potatoes

Sweet potatoes

White flour

White rice

Winter squash (acorn,
  butternut)

Caffeine and Alcohol

Alcoholic beverages

Caffeinated coffee or tea
  (1 cup maximum per day,
  with no other food)

ELIMINATE BAD FATS

Corn oil

Partially hydrogenated
  vegetable oils

Margarine

Shortening

Vegetable oil

JUMP-START
YOUR SUCCESS!

Now that you understand the Sexy Forever nutrition plan, you have all the tools you need to create excellent health, a detoxified body, and the slim figure you have always wanted. The eating program on its own may be enough to get you the results you were hoping for when you picked up this book. That being said, if you are impatient, like most people, you would probably like to have a way to make your results happen both faster and more easily. Faster and easier is pretty appealing!

In this section, I will share with you the tools I have found invaluable to assist in the detoxification and the weight loss process. Select any and all you think may help you break the habits that have been keeping you from being the healthy, slim person you want to become.

As a person who has been at the forefront of the health and wellness field for two decades, I am exposed to just about every product on the market—and every person with a product they'd *like* to be on the market! Those of you who follow me know I am extremely discerning about any products I manufacture or endorse. I demand the highest quality. I expect results. It has to solve a problem for me. If it works for me, I will recommend it to you.

Of the thousands of products I have been asked to review, here are the ones I found worthy of my stamp of approval. Some I manufacture under my own brand and sell at SuzanneSomers.com. For other products, I provide a link to outside websites. And then there are products I encourage you to find at your favorite retail outlet. (You will find these products, or links to these products, at SuzanneSomers.com in the Sexy Forever section, or at the book's companion website, SexyForever.com/book.) Let me share a few of my favorites, from my amazing (if I say so myself) SUZANNE food products to cleansing juices, natural products to curb those derailing cravings, and vitamins and supplements that support detoxification, weight loss, and immune building. Some people want it all, and others are happy to simply follow the nutrition plan. The choice is yours!

SEXY FOREVER MAQUI JUICE BLEND

One of the most effective tools I have found to jump-start the cleansing and weight loss process is this amazing juice. You have spent a lifetime unknowingly building up the toxic burden in your system. With this added first step, you can immediately target the built-up toxins in your cells and release the stored fat.

The amazing maqui berry has a higher concentration of antioxidants than any other known food source on the planet! The high amount of anthocyanins found in the maqui berry give it a rich, deep purple color. They also have an unbelievably great taste. The indigenous Mapuche Indians of the Patagonian region have relied on the maqui berry's benefits for thousands of years. The Patagonian region of South America, specifically in the remote forests of Chile, is one of the most fertile areas on earth. In this region, the maqui berry grows much larger than maqui berries grown elsewhere in the world. While some researchers believe that the maqui berry's high concentration of antioxidants is due to its geographic location, new research theorizes that the reason for the increase in the berry's size and its corresponding nutritional value is the elevated bombardment of ultraviolet rays from a hole in the ozone layer. (Perhaps the only instance where the hole in the ozone layer does anything remotely positive.)

Here are the ingredients included in the Sexy Forever Maqui Juice Blend:

Maqui berry—As we've just read, this main ingredient is an extraordinary source of antioxidants. In addition, it's a leading source of phytochemicals, vitamins A and C, calcium, potassium, iron, and other essential vitamins and minerals.

Aloe vera—This plant is high in vitamins A, C, E, and B, including folic acid and niacin; it also contains minerals including calcium, iron, potassium, magnesium, as well as anti-inflammatory and digestive aids.

Acai berry—The acai berry is high in anthocyanins, Omega-3, 6, and 9 fatty acids, amino acids, protein, a variety of vitamins and minerals, plant sterols, and fiber.

Pomegranate—This is a natural source of vitamins C and B_{12} and potassium.

Mangosteen—This funnily named fruit is valued for its deep purple color and antioxidant properties. It is one of the most popular fruits in Asia.

Noni berry—Rich in fiber, vitamin C, niacin, iron, and potassium.

Goji berry—Contains six essential vitamins, eleven essential minerals, and eighteen amino acids.

Amla fruit—This relatively unknown fruit has one of the highest concentrations of vitamin C of any naturally occurring substance.

Grape skin extract—Contains bioflavonoid and nonbioflavonoid polyphenols. Includes resveratrol, a phytoalexin (type of antibiotic) and polyphenol that is produced naturally by plants when under attack by pathogens such as bacteria or fungi.

Green tea leaf extract—Green tea is a terrific aid in boosting fat loss. It contains a high amount of polyphenols and has been relied on in areas such as Japan, China, India, and Thailand for more than four thousand years.

Pterostilbene—Found in fruits such as blueberries and grapes, this compound has great potential in promoting health. Its benefits rival those of resveratrol.

Gingko biloba extract—By now you've heard of gingko's neuro-protective benefits, which come from its flavonoid glycosides and terpenoids.

The formula for Sexy Forever Maqui Juice Blend supports cleansing and weight management, as well as the immune system and healthy liver function. It is fully loaded with a broad spectrum of antioxidants, phyto-nutrients, polyphenols, and other critical ingredients needed for detoxifi-cation.

For best results, follow the instructions on the bottle to use this prod-uct on Days 1 and 2 of the Detox Phase. You simply mix 16 ounces juice with 16 ounces water and drink it all day long, then repeat for the second day with no other food. The average person sees great results with this amazing jump start! Talk about incentive! Don't be worried that you have to put this fast off until you can commit to being home for two days and chained to your bathroom. It's not that extreme. Yes, you will experience elimination, but in a very controlled manner. Goodbye toxins. Order it on my website, and when it comes in the mail, start the very next morning. For continued antioxidant, cleansing, and weight loss benefits, after you complete the first two days, drink 1 ounce each morning. It's never too early to begin detoxifying your system.

SEXY FOREVER WEIGHT LOSS FORMULA

This scientifically proven weight loss powder includes four clinically tested nutrients (LuraLean, *Phaseolus vulgaris*, irvingia, and green tea phytosome), described on pages 130 to 134, blended together in one formula specifically designed to enhance my Sexy Forever plan. You've read about the science earlier in *Sexy Forever;* now let me give it to you in layman's terms. I will just say that stirring this powder into water and drinking it before your two largest meals of the day literally blasts off the pounds! The clinical studies on these ingredients were proven for weight loss, even when the participants did not alter their eating. Added to the sensible guidelines of my nutrition program and exercise regimen, this gives you a one-two punch that will launch your weight loss with incredible results.

Again, this is available at SuzanneSomers.com under Sexy Forever.

LIFEWAVE NANOTECHNOLOGY PATCHES

I have written at length about David Schmidt and his amazing nanotechnology patches. I encourage you to investigate these products for non-drug solutions to pain, sleep problems, lack of energy, detoxification, and appetite suppression. Here are the two I find particularly beneficial for the topics I have covered in this book.

SP6 Complete Appetite Control Patch

When do those hunger pangs hit you? Afternoon or late-night cravings can sabotage any weight loss plan. This self-adhesive appetite control patch utilizes the ancient principles of acupressure to gently stimulate points on the body that have been used to balance and control appetite for thousands of years. The result is a natural reduction in hunger and food cravings without any drugs, stimulants, or needles entering the body. Plus, the patch is non-transdermal, so nothing enters your body. For people who want appetite suppressants with no stimulants and who don't like to take pills or powders, this makes for a very easy, convenient way to achieve those results.

Y-Age Glutathione Patches

These patches are a safe and natural way to increase the levels of glutathione in the blood. Glutathione, as you've read, is the body's master antioxidant and is crucial to all stages of cellular detoxification. (You can use this patch together with the Appetite Control Patch to maximize your weight-loss results.) I wear this patch most days of the week and feel strongly that it is my best defense against the toxic burden we face daily. These are available at SuzanneSomers.com; click on Lifewave.

Cleansing juice, weight loss powder, patches—so how do you put it all together in a program that works for you? As I have said, with the Sexy Forever plan you have the ability to customize a program to fit your needs. If you cannot afford any of these products, use the eating program alone. If you can swing it, I highly recommend starting on Day 1 and 2 with the cleansing maqui juice. That two-day fast will only require the purchase of one bottle of juice. It really gets things moving! I keep a second bottle and continue to drink 1 ounce per day. Then, every couple of months, I will order an extra bottle and do another 2-day juice fast as a little supercharger. Your choice. I also have had such great results with the weight loss powder. I have my glass of "natural science" before my two largest meals of the day. It just takes the edge off my appetite and activates digestion, fat burning, and metabolism. Imagine the results when you are following Sexy Forever, and supercharging with this scientifically proven, natural formula . . . extraordinary! If you can do it, I would take this product at least through the Level 1—Weight Loss Phase. I am on Level 2 and I still take it. As for the LifeWave patches, I wear the glutathione patch most days of the week for the detoxification benefits, and I add the SP6 patch as needed. Some people will choose the SP6 patch over the powder, because they can put it on and forget about it for the rest of the day. Me? I do it all!

CROSSING THE FINISH LINE: OTHER TOOLS THAT HELP YOU LIVE SEXY FOREVER

In this section I will outline several more products to assist you in stacking the deck for success. Again, each of these lines was created to fill a need, and usually based upon requests from my readers.

When I asked you to give up sugar and artificial sweeteners, you begged me for a recommendation of what to use—this is how All Natural Somer-Sweet was born. When I told you to eat real food without chemicals and preservatives, you asked me to make mealtime easier—this is how the SUZANNE food line was created. When I educated you on the importance of taking vitamins and supplements to replace the vital essentials we are missing, you asked what I take—and this is how RestoreLife Formulas came to be. And when I told you about the toxic chemicals in your skin care and body care products, you asked what you could use instead—and now we have SUZANNE Organics.

None of these products is required for your success; however, they sure make your whole life a whole lot easier. They are all available at Suzanne Somers.com.

RestoreLife Formula Vitamins and Supplements

There are so many brands of vitamins and supplements available at health food, drug, and grocery stores, it can be quite overwhelming for consumers. Plus, the quality of the ingredients can be questionable from some manufacturers. I wanted to make sure the products you choose to take will actually provide you the potency and purity you need to create a positive effect on your health. I work with the highest-quality formulators who insist on only purchasing ingredients from the United States, Europe, and Japan. They have a dedicated scientific board keeping up on the latest, most cutting-edge information to ensure your health is a priority. These are the products I take myself.

All Natural SomerSweet

It looks like sugar, tastes like sugar, bakes like sugar, and now it even measures cup for cup like sugar! All Natural SomerSweet replaces sugar in all your favorite recipes with a blend of 100 percent natural sweeteners you can feel good about using. With a clean, sweet taste, this low-glycemic-index sweetener has 2 grams of fiber per serving and is perfect for anyone with a sweet tooth who is interested in the health benefits of a diet low in sugar.

If you are one of the millions who have enjoyed my Somersize books, you know there are hundreds of recipes calling for my original Somer-Sweet, which was five times sweeter than sugar. All Natural Somer-Sweet has the same sweetness as sugar. To use it instead of original SomerSweet, follow the amounts listed for sugar (or simply take the amount called for original SomerSweet and multiply it by five). If the recipe calls for just SomerSweet, that refers to the original blend. Make sure you calculate the new ratio or your desserts will not be sweet enough.

SUZANNE Desserts

Giving up sugar is no easy task when you first start the program. Once you give up the sugar and white flour, your cravings for sugar and carbohydrates will lessen because you stop that addictive roller coaster of insulin and blood sugar spikes and dives. To help you through the transition, I have a variety of wonderful dessert mixes (again, made with All Natural SomerSweet). Chocolate and Raspberry Mousse, Crème Brûlée, Chocolate Brownie Mix, and more! Some of these dessert mixes are Level 1 and some are Level 2, but all are better choices than a dessert made with sugar. Most of the recipes for these desserts (from scratch) are available in my previous books, and hundreds of recipes are available at SexyForverPlan .com/book, but I also provide these packaged products for convenience.

SUZANNE Seasonings and Sauces

Again, these products are purely for your convenience. Between this book and my series of Somersize books, I have written hundreds of recipes. Anything you could possibly want to eat can be found in these books. For those who don't like to cook from scratch, these delicious products make mealtime a whole lot easier. I select only the highest-quality ingredients. You add the fresh ingredients, and the rest is done for you. My SUZANNE Sea Salt Rubs come in a variety of flavors and turn any piece of meat, poultry, or seafood into a perfectly seasoned entree with the flavors of the most exciting regions of the world. I use Tuscan and Herbs de Provence Sea Salt Rubs several times a week—they're perfect for steaks, chicken, and pork chops. Try the Southwest version for a little kick—great on ribs! I also highly recommend my SUZANNE Simmer Sauces. These are amazing for easy meals in the slow cooker. You add the meat and vegetables and pour on the sauce, which has all the seasoned ingredients measured for you. Beef Bourguignon Simmer Sauce is made with Burgundy, thyme, garlic, olive oil—all the ingredients you would use if you were making it from scratch. Take a simple chuck roast and pour in half a jar of sauce, and in eight hours you have an unbelievably great meal! Try all the varieties for easy, delicious Level 1 meals.

SUZANNE Dips and Salad Dressings

Store-bought versions of these products can be filled with chemicals and preservatives. Usually you will find better options in the refrigerated section—or try these easy mixes and whip up your own in minutes! I have you add the fresh ingredients so I don't have to add those nasty fillers and preservatives. I love the Green Goddess! Yum.

SUZANNE Protein Bars and Shakes

Seriously, these bars and shakes taste like candy bars and milkshakes, but they are made with the highest-quality whey protein (never soy protein) and sweetened with All Natural SomerSweet. These are great choices when you have a hard time finding a meal or snack that works with the program. When Aunt Betty is serving lasagna and you are on Level 1— Weight Loss, keep a bar with you so you don't go hungry or blow it on sugar or white flour. And the protein shakes are so darn good—20 grams of protein per serving and low in sugar and carbohydrates. I love the Orange Cream—tastes like a Creamsicle! Count these products as Protein, Healthy Fats, and 1 serving of Carbohydrates.

SUZANNE Organics Skin Care and Body Care

Once I removed toxins from my diet and household cleaners, I became acutely aware of the products I was continuing to rub on my face and body, all in the name of beauty! I had tried organic products before but had never received the antiaging benefits, so I would slip back to those chemical-based products. As I have said, skin is the largest organ of the body, and if we put toxins on our skin, you can only imagine what we are absorbing transdermally.

I worked with an incredible formulator to develop these products ranging from facial cleansers, toners, and moisturizers to sunless tanning serums, body lotions, and so much more. All are made with natural botanicals for incredible results, in nutrient-rich formulas that truly hydrate the skin. My skin feels better than it has in years. I am so impressed with these products and feel proud to have a line with such integrity and that provides such amazing results.

LET'S GET COOKING: THE RECIPES

When you look through these pages, you will never guess these foods were designed to help you lose weight! The food is loaded with flavor and exciting seasonings to keep you on track. Real food, simply prepared, with the highest-quality ingredients is a gift of life. Use these recipes for breakfasts, soups, salads, starters, vegetables, poultry, meat, and seafood for your amazing and creative meals. And enjoy the fabulous desserts to feel indulged as you shed those pounds.

Each recipe indicates the food groups contained within, to help you as you plan out your meals. Many of the recipes are combinations of Protein, Vegetables, and Healthy Fats that can be combined with other recipes containing any or all of those food groups. You have so much variety and so few restrictions. It's a simple, beautiful way to eat and lose weight.

If you see Carbohydrates in a recipe, remember to count them toward your three servings per day on the Detox Phase, or four servings per day on Level 1—Weight Loss. You will also see Insulin Trigger on recipes that include potatoes, corn, and so on. When you move to Level 2, your body will be able to handle these foods in moderation, so I have given you a handful of recipes for some of my favorites.

In addition, each recipe lists the appropriate phases so you know which recipes to enjoy while you are in Detox, Level 1, or Level 2. If a recipe lists all three phases, it means you may have it during any one of the phases (according to the guidelines you learned about in the previous chapter). If a recipe only lists Level 1 and Level 2, you will not include it during Detox, and can look forward to it when you move to Level 1. Level 2 recipes are to be enjoyed when you reach your goal weight and are living the maintenance lifestyle.

Have fun creating amazing meals, nurturing your precious body, and improving your health and longevity, so you can be Sexy Forever!

Breakfasts

ZUCCHINI AND GREEN TOMATO FRITTATA

Protein, Vegetables, Healthy Fats
Detox, Level 1, Level 2

Serves 6

Eating at home and cooking great meals is one of the joys of life. One day, after picking a zucchini, two green tomatoes, and one heirloom tomato, I made this fantastic frittata!

3 tablespoons extra virgin olive oil
1 onion, chopped
1 zucchini, grated
6 fresh basil leaves, chopped
1 bunch fresh tarragon, chopped
3 sprigs fresh thyme, stems removed
4 eggs, lightly beaten
Sea salt and freshly ground black pepper
½ cup freshly grated Parmesan cheese
3 tomatoes (preferably a mix of green and heirloom), chopped

Preheat the oven to 350 degrees.

Heat a large oven-safe sauté pan on medium high. Add the olive oil and the onion; sauté for about 10 minutes, until browned. Add the zucchini and sauté until brightly colored and tender, about 3 minutes. Add the fresh herbs and the beaten eggs. Season with sea salt and pepper. Leave on the stovetop for 3 minutes to set. Do not stir. Remove from heat and sprinkle with Parmesan cheese. Place in the oven for 10 to 12 minutes, or until center is just set. Slice and serve warm with a side of chopped tomatoes that have been drizzled with olive oil, sea salt, and pepper.

SPICY FRIED EGGS WITH
BASIL AND CRISPY ONIONS

Protein, Vegetables, Healthy Fats
Detox, Level 1, Level 2

Serves 2

As soon as I told my son, Bruce, about the benefits of turmeric, he invented this spicy treat for the morning. He uses a heavy sprinkle of turmeric and cayenne on his fried eggs. It gives a nice antioxidant boost, and your taste buds will say, "Good morning!"

2 large onions
4 tablespoons olive oil
4 large eggs
Sea salt and freshly ground pepper
¼ teaspoon turmeric
⅛ teaspoon cayenne pepper
⅛ teaspoon paprika
4 fresh basil leaves, thinly sliced

To make crispy onions, peel the skin off the onions and slice them as thinly as possible with a sharp knife. In a large skillet, heat 1 tablespoon of olive oil over medium-high heat. When the oil is hot, add the sliced onions. Let them cook until they are brown and crispy, about 10 minutes. Season with salt and pepper. Scrape up the onions with a spatula and divide between two plates.

To fry the eggs, add the remaining 3 tablespoons of olive oil to the same skillet and heat over medium-high. When the oil is nice and hot, crack 2 eggs into the skillet. Sprinkle with salt, pepper, turmeric, cayenne, and paprika. Cook until the whites start to brown on the edges. Cover the skillet with a lid and cook for 1 minute longer. When you lift the lid, the whites will be cooked all the way through and the yolks will be slightly runny. If you prefer them more cooked, leave the lid on longer. Lift the eggs out with a spatula and place onto the plated onions. Repeat with the other 2 eggs. Top with fresh basil and serve.

PEACH RASPBERRY FRUIT SMOOTHIE

Fruit
Detox, Level 1, Level 2

Serves 2

I love starting my mornings with a fruit smoothie! For an icy frozen treat, use frozen fruit or add a handful of ice.

2 cups frozen peaches
1 cup frozen raspberries
¾ cup guava juice

Place the fruit and juice into a blender and process until smooth. Adjust the amount of juice to create the consistency you prefer.

TROPICAL FRUIT SMOOTHIE

Fruit
Detox, Level 1, Level 2

Serves 2

A taste of the islands . . . delicious! There is a brand of juice called Ceres that has a line of exotic flavors and no added sugars. Of course, you may use any brand, just watch for added sugar. Use fresh or frozen fruit; I have specified frozen only because these exotic fruits can be hard to find in some areas.

  2 cups frozen mango
  1 cup frozen pineapple
  ¾ cup passion fruit juice

Place the fruit and juice into a blender and process until smooth. Adjust the amount of juice to create the consistency you prefer.

🌿 BERRY POWER SMOOTHIE 🌿

Fruit
Detox, Level 1, Level 2

Serves 2

Packed with antioxidants, these berries start your day off right! Either fresh or frozen work well.

1 cup frozen blueberries
1 cup frozen raspberries
1 cup frozen blackberries
¾ cup cherry juice

Place the fruit and juice into a blender and process until smooth. Adjust the amount of juice to create the consistency you prefer.

🌿 BREAKFAST QUINOA 🌿

Carbohydrates
Detox, Level 1, Level 2

Serves 2

Quinoa (pronounced "keen-wha") is a very versatile grain. It's related to the leafy green family, with a low glycemic index (about the same as wild rice), so it gives you the satisfaction of a carbohydrate without the same consequences. And it has the nutrients of a complete protein! I use it as a side dish at dinner, or as a main dish as a pilaf, but here's a truly novel idea—breakfast! Instead of oatmeal I have quinoa with goat milk and a little agave for sweetness. Gluten free, dairy free, sugar free, and delicious.

1 cup quinoa
2 cups water
¼ teaspoon sea salt
Goat milk (or nonfat milk)
Agave nectar

In a small saucepan, combine quinoa, water, and salt. Bring to a boil, then cover and decrease the heat to low and cook for 15 minutes. The water should be completely evaporated. Fluff with a fork and place into serving bowls. Add a splash of goat milk and a squeeze of agave.

Soups, Salads, and Appetizers

SPRING VEGETABLE AND TURKEY SOUP

. . . .

Protein, Vegetables, Healthy Fats, Insulin Triggers
Level 2

Serves 8

Your immune system will turn backflips with joy when you eat this fresh, delicious soup. The antioxidant-rich fresh vegetables keep their crunch, because rather than being boiled with the broth, they are grilled or quickly pan-fried, then added to the broth at the last minute, with freshly sliced turkey. Feel free to use chicken instead of turkey. And for a Detox or Level 1 option, omit the wine, corn, and carrots.

    1 turkey breast, on the bone
    4 turkey wings
    Extra virgin olive oil
    1 tablespoon SUZANNE Herbs de Provence Sea Salt Rub (or any
        other brand)
    1 cup white wine
    12 cups chicken broth
    6 ears fresh corn
    1 bunch asparagus
    4 leeks
    8 stalks celery
    6 carrots
    2 cups sugar snap peas
    1 bunch fresh flat-leaf parsley, finely chopped

Preheat the oven to 350 degrees.

Rub the turkey breast and wings generously with olive oil and the Herbs de Provence. Pour the wine into the bottom of a roasting pan and add the turkey. Loosely tent the meat with foil. Roast until the internal temperature of the breast reaches 160 degrees when measured with a meat thermometer. Remove the foil and continue roasting until the internal temperature reaches 180 degrees. The cooking time will vary, depending upon the size of the turkey breast.

Cut the breast meat off the bone and set aside, covered in foil to keep warm. Save the roasted breast bone for your next batch of homemade broth. If using store-bought broth, add those bones to the broth to make it richer.

Place the broth in a soup pot on medium-high heat and bring to a boil. Add the cooked turkey wings to add extra flavor.

Meanwhile, husk and clean the corn and place them on a hot grill, turning frequently to brown all sides. Remove from the grill and set aside to cool. Slice the kernels off the cob. Add the cobs to the broth.

Trim the tough ends from the asparagus. Toss onto the hot grill, turning frequently to lightly char on all sides. Remove and chop into bite-size pieces.

Wash the leeks well. Trim the tough dark green ends and add them to the broth. Finely chop the white and light green parts and set aside. Chop the celery and carrots, adding any trimmed ends to the soup pot. String the snap peas and chop into bite-size pieces.

Place a large sauté pan on high heat. Add olive oil, then the chopped leeks, celery, carrots, and snap peas. Sauté for 3 to 4 minutes, until bursting with bright colors. Add the grilled corn and asparagus and stir to combine.

Strain the broth into another soup pot. Ladle into serving bowls and add chopped pieces of turkey, a generous serving of tender, sautéed vegetables, and a garnish of chopped parsley.

🌿 MIKRI GREEK SALAD 🌿

Protein, Vegetables, Healthy Fats
Detox, Level 1, Level 2

Serves 4

When tomatoes are ripened on the vine, we eat them constantly. If you are used to tasteless tomatoes from the supermarket, it's because they are picked when they are green and ripened with ethylene. Look for locally grown tomatoes at farmer's markets, or plant a few seeds of your own. Our organic gardener gave us this tip—pour your leftover coffee with added milk and sugar over them. They thrive! Greek salads are easy to throw together and always please. This one is made with sweet little cherry tomatoes—that's why it's called Mikri ("small" in Greek). With a small dice on the cucumber and onion, it's more like a salsa. This is what my daughter-in-law, Caroline, made to garnish those awesome Lamb Carnitas (page 267).

2 pints organic cherry tomatoes
3 Persian cucumbers (or pickling cucumbers), cut into ¼-inch dice
½ medium red onion, cut into ¼-inch dice
Sea salt and freshly ground black pepper
4 tablespoons extra virgin olive oil
Juice from ½ lemon
8 ounces feta cheese, crumbled
Fresh oregano leaves, finely chopped

Slice the tomatoes in half and combine with the diced cucumber and red onion. Season with sea salt and pepper. Just before serving, gently toss with the olive oil and a squeeze of lemon. Sprinkle with crumbled feta and garnish with a generous pinch of fresh oregano.

🌿 HUMMUS ON FIRE 🌿

··

Carbohydrates, Vegetables, Healthy Fats
Level 1, Level 2

Serves 4

I love hummus as an appetizer with fresh vegetables. This recipe is like hummus on steroids. It's loaded with extra spices, full of antioxidants, to make it a superfood! Turmeric gives it a fabulous orange color, and cayenne gives it a red color and the kick of spice. This is fabulous with the Lamb Carnitas (page 267). Count this dish as a Carbohydrate.

4 cups cooked or canned garbanzo beans (chickpeas), drained
3 garlic cloves
4 tablespoons lemon juice
2 tablespoons tahini (sesame paste)
2 tablespoons extra virgin olive oil
½ teaspoon cayenne
2 teaspoons turmeric
2 sprigs fresh parsley
Sea salt and freshly ground black pepper

Combine all the ingredients in a food processor and process until well combined. Taste and add more lemon juice and seasoning as needed.

🌿 BASIL PARSLEY PESTO 🌿

••

Protein, Vegetables, Healthy Fats, Carbohydrates
Detox, Level 1, Level 2

Makes about 1 cup

This is the best pesto I have ever tasted in my life. Maybe it's because I grow my own basil, so it's that much fresher. Or maybe it's the pride I take in it that makes it taste so good! Every summer I make batches of this pesto and freeze it in small containers. When freezing, I do not add the Parmesan. It tastes much better if you add it when you are ready to use the pesto. I use this in soups, stuffed under chicken skin, on salads, on tomatoes with mozzarella, and of course over pasta on occasion. When basil is in season, buy as much as you can afford and make your own batches. You will have it all through the winter if you do, and it always zips up a great dish. Count the small amount of pine nuts in this recipe toward your Carbohydrate intake.

2 cups basil leaves, loosely packed
½ cup flat-leaf parsley, loosely packed
½ cup freshly grated Parmesan cheese (see Note)
¼ cup toasted pine nuts
¾ cup extra virgin olive oil
1 clove garlic, minced
½ teaspoon sea salt
Freshly ground black pepper

Set aside a small bowl filled with ice water. Bring a small pot of water to a boil and add the basil leaves for 30 seconds to soften. Remove immediately and plunge the leaves into the ice water. After 30 to 60 seconds, remove the leaves from the ice bath, squeeze out the excess water, and place into a food processor. Add the remaining ingredients and puree until smooth.

Note: If freezing, omit the Parmesan and add after you defrost it.

GRILLED TOMATOES
WITH CREAMY BURRATA

Vegetables, Healthy Fats
Detox, Level 1, Level 2

Serves 4

Nothing is more delicious than freshly picked tomatoes. My favorites are vine-ripened heirloom varieties. Try a farmer's market for just-picked freshness. I grow my own tomatoes, and some years I have a better crop than others; these little guys have their temperaments, just like women! In this recipe, they are grilled, which changes the flavor and chars them in the most delicious way. Serve with creamy burrata cheese and you will be stunned by how tasty they are.

4 ripe tomatoes
8 ounces burrata cheese (or fresh mozzarella), sliced
Extra virgin olive oil
Sea salt and freshly ground black pepper
Basil Parsley Pesto, for garnish (page 221)

Preheat a grill to high. Place the whole tomatoes onto the grill and cook, turning occasionally, until the skin is wrinkled but not bursting, 3 to 5 minutes. The time will vary depending upon the size of the tomatoes. Remove from the heat and place each tomato onto a serving plate. Divide the burrata among the plates. Drizzle olive oil over the tomato and cheese, then season with sea salt and pepper. Garnish with a dollop of basil pesto.

GRILLED FENNEL AND WATERCRESS SALAD

Vegetables, Healthy Fats
Level 1, Level 2

Serves 4

Imagine the intensity of flavor in this dish . . . it's alive with the licorice of the fennel, the sweetness of the grilled oranges, and the sea salt to balance. Fresh and tasty, this easy-to-make dish makes a great salad all year long. I love this with pan-fried sole for a lovely, light dinner. Using the orange creates a small sugar imbalance. I would not recommend this for Detox, but if you are doing well on Level 1, you are fine to include the small amount of orange.

2 bunches fresh watercress (or arugula), trimmed
4 fennel bulbs, sliced ¼ inch thick (reserve the fronds for garnish)
Extra virgin olive oil
2 oranges, cut in half
Sea salt and freshly ground black pepper

Preheat a grill to medium heat.

Place the watercress onto a serving plate and set aside. Brush the fennel with olive oil and place onto the grill with the oranges, flesh side down. Grill the fennel until nicely browned and tender, about 3 minutes. Remove the fennel and oranges from the grill. Place the grilled fennel onto the bed of watercress, then squeeze the grilled oranges over the top. Drizzle with a little olive oil, season with sea salt and pepper, and garnish with fennel fronds.

ARUGULA SALAD
🌿 WITH GOAT CHEESE AND 🌿
PERSIAN CUCUMBER

Vegetables, Healthy Fats
Detox, Level 1, Level 2

Serves 4

Fresh, bountiful, delicious, and takes no time to whip up. Persian cucumbers have a much better taste than their thick-skinned American counterparts. They are long and thin and do not need peeling. If you can't find them, pickling cucumbers also make a good choice.

> 6 Persian cucumbers
> 1 pint cherry tomatoes
> 1 shallot, minced
> Sea salt and freshly ground black pepper
> Juice of ½ lemon
> 8 fresh basil leaves
> ½ pound arugula
> Extra virgin olive oil
> 6 ounces goat cheese

Quarter each cucumber lengthwise, then thinly slice into bite-size pieces and place into a bowl. Quarter the cherry tomatoes and add to the bowl. Add the minced shallot, sea salt, pepper, and a squeeze of lemon. Toss gently. Stack 4 of the basil leaves, then roll and thinly slice into a chiffonade. Sprinkle over the tomatoes. Place the arugula into a bowl and lightly toss with olive oil, then season with sea salt and pepper. Place a bed of arugula onto serving plates, then top with the tomato and cucumbers. Slice the goat cheese into 4 equal pieces and add one to each plate. Garnish with a basil leaf.

ROASTED PEPPERS AND OLIVES

Vegetables, Healthy Fats, Carbohydrates
Detox, Level 1, Level 2

Serves 4

This is so simple and delicious, but sometimes it's the simple dishes that linger in our memories. The peppers are slightly crunchy and yummy tossed with a splash of sweet balsamic vinegar. This makes a beautiful salad on its own, or a lively side dish to bring a simple piece of meat, poultry, or fish to life. Remember to count the olives toward your Carbohydrates.

2 red bell peppers
2 orange bell peppers
2 yellow bell peppers
Extra virgin olive oil
10 black olives
10 green olives
1 tablespoon capers, drained
1 tablespoon balsamic vinegar
Sea salt and freshly ground black pepper

Preheat a grill to medium. Slice the peppers in half lengthwise. Remove the seeds and spines. Cut each half of the flesh into about 4 good-sized pieces so they will not fall through the slots of the grill. Place the peppers on the grill and cook, turning frequently, until nicely browned, about 4 minutes. Remove from the heat and place in a bowl. Toss with olive oil, the olives, capers, balsamic vinegar, sea salt, and pepper. Serve warm.

🌿 CHOPPED ANTIPASTO SALAD 🌿

Protein, Vegetables, Healthy Fats
Detox, Level 1, Level 2

Serves 2

Wild arugula, celery leaves, and escarole give you a burst of antioxidants with their dark green leafy goodness. Wild arugula has a lovely ragged edge and slightly bitter taste. The idea to use the celery leaves came from growing celery in my garden. I had so many gorgeous leaves that are normally trimmed off by the time a head of celery gets to the grocery store. Instead, I chopped up the leaves and added them to the salad. Delicious and packed with nutrition! Escarole is an underused lettuce with a hearty texture. Top with grilled chicken covered in herbs and plenty of Italian additions. You have a salad worth staying at home for—for lunch or dinner!

Herb-Grilled Chicken Breasts
    2 boneless, skinless chicken breasts
    Extra virgin olive oil
    Sea salt and freshly ground black pepper
    1 teaspoon dried rosemary
    1 teaspoon dried thyme
    1 teaspoon dried basil
    2 teaspoons paprika

Antipasto Salad
    ½ head escarole leaves (about 4 cups)
    8 ounces arugula
    2 large handfuls chopped celery leaves (about 1 cup)
    3 stalks celery, chopped
    1 cup grated mozzarella cheese
    1 vine-ripened tomato, chopped

½ cup marinated artichoke hearts

½ cup sliced hearts of palm

¼ cup sliced pepperoncini

Red Wine Vinaigrette

½ cup extra virgin olive oil

2 tablespoons red wine vinegar

Sea salt and freshly ground black pepper

Dash of sesame oil (optional)

Drizzle the chicken breasts with oil. Season with salt, pepper, and the dried herbs and paprika until well coated on both sides. Grill on medium-high heat, about 4 minutes per side, until cooked through. Set aside to cool. Chop into bite-size pieces.

Assemble the salad ingredients in a large bowl. Whisk together the vinaigrette ingredients in a small bowl. Pour over the salad and toss. Drizzle a touch of sesame oil over the top and toss again. Add the reserved chicken and give one final toss. Taste for seasoning and adjust. Place into salad bowls and serve.

Vegetables

🌿 GRILLED ZUCCHINI 🌿

Vegetables, Healthy Fats, Carbohydrates
Level 1, Level 2

Serves 4

For most of the year, zucchini grows like crazy in the warm California sun where we live. It's most tender if you catch it at about 1 ½ inches in circumference. You can blink and it will be 4 inches thick! I pick several each day from my organic garden, and I'm always looking for new ways to cook it. This recipe combines the tart taste of plain yogurt with fresh dill and lemon. Yogurt is listed as a Carbohydrate, so count a little toward your servings. For a version with no carbs, use a basil pesto instead of the yogurt and dill.

    4 ounces plain whole-milk yogurt, preferably Greek style
    2 tablespoons freshly chopped dill, or 2 teaspoons dried
    Extra virgin olive oil
    Juice of 1 lemon
    Sea salt and freshly ground black pepper
    4 medium zucchini, sliced ½ inch thick

Preheat a grill to medium high. In a small bowl, mix together the yogurt, dill, 1 tablespoon olive oil, the lemon juice, and sea salt and pepper. Add the sliced zucchini and gently stir until the zucchini is well coated.

Place the zucchini on the grill and cook until browned on both sides, about 3 minutes per side. Serve immediately.

🌿 CARAMELIZED FENNEL 🌿

Vegetables, Healthy Fats
Detox, Level 1, Level 2

Serves 4

Fennel grows abundantly in our organic garden. I love the fresh, crisp taste. Our grandkids like to chew on the stalks while we are walking up the hill back to the house. I usually chop it into salads. Last week I had soooo much of it, Alan and I had a hard time eating it all. I decided to cook it down in olive oil and butter, and the result was divine! Slow-cooked and incredibly sweet as it caramelizes. All those nutrients? A bonus!

2 tablespoons olive oil
2 tablespoons organic unsalted butter
6 fennel bulbs, trimmed and thinly sliced
Salt and freshly ground black pepper

Place a large sauté pan over medium-high heat. Add the olive oil and butter. When melted, add the sliced fennel and sauté for about 10 minutes, turning consistently for even browning. When brown on all sides, reduce heat to low, cover, and continue cooking for another 10 minutes, until tender when pierced with a fork. Season with salt and pepper.

SAUTÉED BOK CHOY

Vegetables, Healthy Fats

Detox, Level 1, Level 2

Serves 4

My husband grew up in an interesting household: his mother ran a boardinghouse and seventeen people lived with him his entire life, including seven Chinese brothers with whom he became very close. I grew up in an Irish household where my mother cooked meat and potatoes, whereas Alan was exposed to winter melon, water chestnuts, and exotic vegetables like bok choy. Bok choy tastes great in soup, sautéed, or eaten raw in a salad. These are tender and sweet from the soy sauce.

3 tablespoons extra virgin olive oil
4 heads bok choy, quartered lengthwise
2 tablespoons soy sauce
¼ teaspoon white pepper

Place a medium sauté pan over medium-high heat. When hot, add the olive oil, then the bok choy. Sauté for about 6 minutes, until wilted and tender. Add the soy sauce and white pepper. Stir to combine. Serve immediately.

BROILED BELGIAN ENDIVE
WITH PARMESAN

Vegetables, Healthy Fats
Detox, Level 1, Level 2

Serves 4

Belgian endive is sautéed until soft, then broiled with Parmesan until hot and bubbly. It takes on a whole other flavor when cooked like this.

3 tablespoons extra virgin olive oil
4 heads Belgian endive, halved lengthwise
Sea salt and freshly ground black pepper
½ cup freshly grated Parmesan cheese

Move a rack to the top position in the oven and turn the broiler to high.

Place an oven-safe sauté pan over high heat. When hot, add the olive oil, then the Belgian endive. Season with sea salt and pepper. Cook for 2 to 3 minutes per side, carefully turning with a spatula. When soft and lightly browned, remove from the heat. Turn endive cut side up and sprinkle with the Parmesan. Place the pan under the hot broiler, watching carefully, for 1 to 2 minutes, until the cheese is bubbling. Serve immediately.

🌿 SAUTÉED KALE 🌿

··

Vegetables, Healthy Fats
Detox, Level 1, Level 2

Serves 4

Kale is considered a superfood because it is so nutrient dense. In fact, it's nearly twice as packed with phytochemicals as the second-highest-rated vegetable. While it's quite bitter raw, it gets sweet and delicious when sautéed. Try it!

3 tablespoons olive oil
1 yellow onion, chopped
4 bunches kale, chopped
1 tablespoon butter, optional
Sea salt and freshly ground black pepper

Place a large sauté pan over medium-high heat and add the olive oil. Add the onion and sauté until nicely browned, 10 to 15 minutes. Add the kale and sauté until the leaves are soft and wilted, 7 to 10 minutes. Swirl in the butter until well distributed, then season with sea salt and pepper. Serve warm.

🌿 SAUTÉED BROCCOLI FLORETS 🌿

Vegetables, Healthy Fats
Detox, Level 1, Level 2

Serves 4

Broccoli is another fabulous superfood for cancer prevention. Ounce for ounce, broccoli has more vitamin C than oranges, as much calcium as milk, and three times the fiber of a slice of wheat-bran bread, and it's one of the richest sources of vitamin A in the whole produce section! Some people don't like steamed broccoli, so to get all of those important nutrients, try it another way. In this recipe the broccoli is chopped into very small bites and sautéed in butter and sea salt to coat each piece. Amazing.

1 large head broccoli
1 tablespoon olive oil
1 tablespoon butter (optional)
Sea salt and freshly ground black pepper

Wash and trim off all but 1 inch of the stem of the broccoli. Chop the remaining stem and broccoli tops into tiny bites, about ¼-inch pieces. Sauté over medium-high heat in the olive oil and butter until bright green and tender. Season with sea salt and black pepper.

SAUTÉED MUSHROOMS AND ONIONS

Vegetables, Healthy Fats
Detox, Level 1, Level 2

Serves 4

These mushrooms taste great with chicken or steak. Plus, you'll benefit from iron, zinc, fiber, essential amino acids, and a host of vitamins and minerals! White- and brown-colored vegetables are particularly good for lowering blood pressure and cholesterol.

2 tablespoons olive oil
2 onions, thinly sliced
4 cups mushrooms (shiitake, oyster, or button), chopped
1 tablespoon fresh thyme leaves (or 1 teaspoon dried)
2 tablespoons butter (optional)
Sea salt and freshly ground black pepper

Place a large sauté pan over medium heat and add the olive oil. Add the onions and sauté until caramelized, about 30 minutes. Turn the heat to medium high and add the mushrooms and thyme. Sauté until the mushrooms are crisp on the edges, about 15 minutes. Stir in the butter and swirl until melted. Season with sea salt and black pepper.

BROILED RADICCHIO
WITH PROSCIUTTO

Protein, Vegetables, Healthy Fats
Detox, Level 1, Level 2

Serves 4

Hot radicchio, wrapped in prosciutto, then cooked under the broiler, is salty and earthy. This is a wonderful first course or side dish. My husband asks for it all the time.

2 heads radicchio, halved
Extra virgin olive oil
Sea salt and freshly ground black pepper
Fresh basil pesto
4 thin slices prosciutto

Preheat the oven to 350 degrees.

Drizzle the cut sides of the radicchio with olive oil, then season with sea salt and pepper. Place on a baking sheet and roast for 15 minutes, until soft and golden. Remove the baking sheet from the oven and set aside.

Carefully move the rack to the top position in the oven. Turn the broiler to high.

Brush the roasted radicchio with pesto, then lay a slice of prosciutto across the top. Broil until the prosciutto is golden brown and crispy. Serve immediately.

GRILLED ARTICHOKES
AND LEMONS

Vegetables, Healthy Fats
Detox, Level 1, Level 2

Serves 2

My husband has never liked artichokes; this is particularly disappointing because I grow them. They are not only beautiful plants, but are so delicious and are loaded with great nutrients. I'd tried every way possible to cook and prepare artichokes and he still didn't like them . . . until I did them this way. If you make them you too will get oohs and ahhs and a dish that's lick-your-fingers scrumptious. A half was not enough for him; therefore I am suggesting one per person. They are also great as leftovers the next day.

2 artichokes
Extra virgin olive oil
5 fresh lemons, halved
Sea salt

Place a large pot of salted water to boil on the stovetop. Trim the outer leaves from the artichokes and cut them in half lengthwise. Scoop out the choke. When the water is boiling, add the artichoke halves and parboil until tender, 15 to 20 minutes. Meanwhile, heat a grill to medium. Pierce the artichokes with a fork to check for doneness. They should be tender but still firm. When done, remove them from the water and drizzle them with olive oil, then squeeze the juice from 1 lemon on all sides, and season with sea salt.

(continued)

Place the artichokes, cut side down, onto the grill for about 7 minutes, turning to cook all sides. Place additional lemon halves on the grill, cut side down. When the artichokes are nicely browned, remove them and the grilled lemons. Squeeze juice from the grilled lemons over the artichokes, then drizzle a little more olive oil over each and sprinkle with sea salt. Serve immediately.

🌿 GRILLED GUACAMOLE 🌿

Vegetables, Healthy Fats, Carbohydrates
Level 1, Level 2

Serves 8

Grilled avocados? I know! It is as unusual-sounding as it is delicious. Try it and you might find yourself saying, "Holy guacamole." This is amazing served with Southwest Roasted Chicken (page 256). Since avocados have carbohydrates, you may enjoy about ½ cup of this on Level 1, according to the plan guidelines for Carbs.

    4 avocados, halved
    ½ red onion
    2 ripe tomatoes (preferably heirloom), chopped
    1 clove garlic, minced
    Juice of 1 lime
    Extra virgin olive oil
    Sea salt and freshly ground black pepper

Preheat a grill to medium high. Halve and pit the avocados. Place avocados (flesh side down) and the onion half onto the grill. Grill the avocados for about 2 minutes, then remove them from the heat and scoop the flesh into a small bowl. Grill the onion for about 5 minutes. Remove from the heat, then chop and add to the avocados. Add the chopped tomatoes, garlic, lime juice, and a drizzle of olive oil. Season with sea salt and pepper. Gently mix together and serve.

ROASTED
BUTTERNUT SQUASH

Healthy Fats, Insulin Triggers
Level 2

Serves 4

Butternut squash is sweet and delicious, and loaded with beta carotene—a wonderful antioxidant, particularly good for healthy eyes and skin. Great for Level 2, since it's an Insulin Trigger.

1 large butternut squash
Extra virgin olive oil
½ stick butter
Sea salt and freshly ground black pepper

Preheat the oven to 350 degrees.

Cut the squash in half lengthwise and remove the seeds. Drizzle with olive oil. Place the squash halves in a shallow roasting pan or on a baking sheet with the cut sides facing up. Pour ¼ cup water in the bottom of the pan. Gently cover with foil and bake until the squash is easily pierced with a fork, about 45 minutes. Remove from the oven. When cool enough to handle, scoop the flesh into a bowl (discard the skin). Add the butter to the squash, plus sea salt and pepper. Puree with a fork or a masher until smooth. Taste and add more butter, salt, and pepper, if desired.

✷ LIME CORN ✷

Healthy Fats, Insulin Triggers
Level 2

Serves 4

My husband loves corn, Insulin Trigger or not! We grow it in Palm Springs in our organic vegetable garden. He lovingly monitors its growth, awaiting the day when it's finally ready to eat. The first few ears get peeled and eaten on-site. They never even make it up the hill to the house. Then he allows me to "have my way" with them. This is a perfectly simple and delicious way to prepare fresh corn. The taste of the grilled kernels with butter and salt is wonderful. And the lime really brightens the flavor. Just remember to reserve this treat for Level 2.

4 ears fresh corn, husks on
Extra virgin olive oil
4 tablespoons (½ stick) butter, melted
Sea salt and freshly ground black pepper
Juice of 2 limes

Soak the corn in their husks in salted water for 1 hour prior to grilling. Heat a grill to high. Pull the husks back (or off, if desired) and place the corn on the grill. Brush the corn with olive oil and grill, turning frequently, for about 5 minutes. Remove from the heat and serve with melted butter, sea salt, and pepper. Add a squeeze of fresh lime juice to each ear before serving.

🌿 BAKED YAMS 🌿

. . . .

Healthy Fats, Insulin Triggers
Level 2

Serves 4

Some people only associate yams with the canned style often served at the holidays with marshmallows on top. You will also love them freshly baked like this! Plus, you'll be getting vitamin C, potassium, manganese, fiber, and vitamin B_6. Yams are a wonderful heart-healthy vegetable with beta-carotene for healthy eyes and skin. Enjoy them on Level 2.

4 yams
4 tablespoons butter
Sea salt and freshly ground black pepper

Wash the yams and pierce them in several places with a fork. Place on a baking sheet lined with parchment or foil and bake at 350 degrees for 60 to 80 minutes or until a fork easily pierces through the skin to the center. Remove from the oven and slice in half lengthwise. Mash the inside of the yam with a fork, adding the butter, sea salt, and freshly ground black pepper. Serve warm.

SMASHED YUKON GOLD POTATOES

Healthy Fats, Insulin Triggers
Level 2

Serves 4

My son, Bruce, perfected this recipe. One night when he was home with the girls, they baked potatoes, then smashed them with a mallet and rebaked them, drizzled with olive oil and sea salt. What a "smash" hit! Everyone loved them. Both of my granddaughters are allergic to gluten, so potatoes come in handy at their house. For the rest of us, it's an extraordinary treat for Level 2—and a reward for getting your cells cleaned out. Yukon gold potatoes have a wonderful buttery flavor, but if you can't find them, any potato will do.

4 Yukon gold potatoes
Extra virgin olive oil
Sea salt and freshly ground black pepper

Preheat the oven to 350 degrees. Pierce the potatoes with a fork in several spots. When the oven is hot, place the washed, wet potatoes onto a baking sheet and bake for 1 hour, until the skin is crusty. Carefully smash each potato with a mallet until each is about 1 inch thick. Drizzle olive oil over each potato, then season liberally with sea salt and pepper. Return them to the oven and cook for 25 minutes more. Serve immediately.

ASPARAGUS JALAPEÑO RISOTTO

Vegetables, Healthy Fats, Insulin Triggers
Level 2

Serves 4 to 6

We don't eat much white rice in our house, but I do love a good risotto every now and then. Alan is gluten intolerant, so a delicious rice dish is a real treat for him. I am predominantly drawn to Italian food, particularly Tuscan food, but I branched out the other night and did a roasted chicken with SUZANNE Southwest Sea Salt Rub and came up with this risotto on the spot to go with it. It has a little bit of jalapeño, but if you only use one chile it's not spicy at all—just flavorful. If you like more of a kick, increase the jalapeño or use a hotter chile, like a serrano. Obviously, this is a Level 2 meal because of the rice.

2 to 3 tablespoons extra virgin olive oil
½ red onion, diced
3 cloves garlic, minced
1 jalapeño, diced
1 cup arborio rice
4 to 5 cups chicken broth
1 bunch asparagus, chopped into ½-inch pieces

Place a large sauté pan over medium-high heat. Add the olive oil and red onion and sauté until the onion is translucent, about 5 minutes. Add the garlic and jalapeño and continue to sauté for another 10 minutes, until the onion is browned and the jalapeño is tender. Add the rice and toss with the oil, onion, and jalapeño mixture until well coated and the rice just begins to turn golden.

Add 1 cup of broth and stir until it is absorbed by the rice. Add the next cup of broth and stir until absorbed. Add the third cup of broth and the chopped asparagus. The asparagus will cook as the broth is absorbed. Add the fourth cup of broth, making sure to test the rice for doneness. Risotto should be served al dente and "brothy," so don't let all the broth be absorbed. If the rice is still not cooked, add 1 more cup of broth.

CARAMELIZED CUMIN CARROTS

Healthy Fats, Insulin Triggers
Level 2

Serves 4

The rather exotic flavor of these caramelized carrots will surprise you. The cumin and cayenne are balanced by the sweetness of the agave for a delicious candied treat.

> 3 tablespoons olive oil
> 3 tablespoons cumin
> 1 teaspoon cayenne
> ¼ cup agave nectar
> 4 carrots, sliced ¼ inch thick on the diagonal
> Sea salt and freshly ground black pepper

In a small bowl, combine the olive oil, cumin, cayenne, and agave.

Place a large sauté pan over medium heat and add a dash of olive oil to cover the bottom of the pan. Add the carrots and sauté for 2 to 3 minutes, until bright orange and just releasing their flavor. Add the agave mixture to the carrots and gently sauté to coat all the carrots. Season with sea salt and pepper. Sauté for an additional 10 minutes, until the carrots become brown and caramelized. Stir constantly, and watch the heat: if the agave starts to burn, lower the heat. Serve immediately.

Poultry, Fish, and Meat

CHICKEN DRUMSTICKS WITH LEMON SLICES AND CRISPY HERBS

Protein, Vegetables, Healthy Fats
Detox, Level 1, Level 2

Serves 6

Think of this as your go-to Tuesday night dinner *and* Wednesday's lunch. I make a dozen just for me and Al, and we sit at our computers the next day and eat them cold for lunch. We are far more glamorous than you realize! The grandkids really love these drumsticks, too . . . they are simply good, and fun to eat. I like to smother them with freshly chopped garlic and herbs from my garden. You may use any combination of fresh herbs; I usually ask the grand-kids to surprise me, but my favorite herb with chicken is fresh thyme. The roasted lemon slices are incredible! The rind gets very soft and candied and tastes great with each bite of chicken.

12 chicken drumsticks
Extra virgin olive oil
Sea salt and freshly ground black pepper
10 cloves fresh garlic, minced
3 to 5 cups loosely packed fresh herbs, stems discarded (thyme, rosemary, tarragon, sage, or parsley)
3 lemons, cut into thin slices

Preheat the oven to 350 degrees.

Place the drumsticks in a large roasting pan. Generously drizzle them with olive oil, then season with sea salt, pepper, and the garlic and fresh herbs. Place the lemon slices on top of each drumstick and the leftovers in the bottom of the pan. Place the pan in the oven and cook for about 80 minutes. While roasting, turn the drumsticks and scrape the lemon slices from the bottom of the pan from time to time to loosen and evenly brown. Serve the drumsticks with the cooked lemon slices and crispy herbs.

🌿 ROASTED TURMERIC CHICKEN 🌿

....

Protein, Vegetables, Healtovy Fats
Detox, Level 1, Level 2

Serves 6

I love how a roasted chicken makes the whole house smell; it feels comforting and safe. Anyone can roast a chicken. It's easy to do and delicious. Plus you can make a chicken last a week by using leftovers for chicken salad and the carcass for chicken soup. Chicken is already a great food, but adding the turmeric turns it into a superfood!

> Extra virgin olive oil
> 3 tablespoons turmeric
> One 5-pound roasting chicken
> Sea salt and freshly ground black pepper
> 1 bunch fresh thyme, leaves only
> 1 bunch fresh sage, leaves only
> 4 tablespoons butter
> 1 cup chicken broth, preferably homemade (see page 260)

Preheat the oven to 350 degrees.

Make a paste with the olive oil and turmeric. Place the chicken in a roasting pan and brush on the paste, covering the entire chicken until it is a beautiful orange color. Sprinkle liberally with sea salt and pepper, then scatter the fresh herbs over the top. Dot with half of the butter. Roast for about 1 hour and 20 minutes (about 20 minutes per pound). The skin should be golden and crispy.

To make a quick gravy out of the pan drippings, remove the chicken and herbs from the pan and place on a cutting board. Pour most of the fat out of the roasting pan, reserving about 1 tablespoon. Place the pan on the stovetop over high heat. Add the chicken broth and scrape the browned bits from the bottom of the pan. Continue to boil until the liquid is reduced by half. Turn off the heat, then add the remaining butter and swirl until combined and smooth.

Carve the chicken, and serve with a spoonful of pan gravy and a sprinkle of herbs.

CILANTRO GINGER
LEMON CHICKEN

....

Protein, Vegetables, Healthy Fats
Detox, Level 1, Level 2

Serves 4 to 6

Packed with flavor and antioxidants, this dish puts the typical boring chicken dinner to shame! Thanks to garlic, ginger, chiles, cayenne, coriander, turmeric, and fresh lemon juice, this super chicken is a superfood. This is great with brown basmati rice, if you choose to have Carbohydrates with it.

¼ cup extra virgin olive oil
2 pounds chicken legs and thighs, skinless
Sea salt and white pepper
8 cloves garlic, finely chopped
2 tablespoons finely chopped fresh ginger
½ serrano chile, seeded and finely chopped
¼ teaspoon cayenne pepper
2 teaspoons ground coriander
2 teaspoons turmeric
2 bunches cilantro, leaves only
Juice of 2 lemons
1 cup water

Add the olive oil to a large sauté or braising pan (choose a pan with a lid as you'll need it later) and heat over medium high. Season the chicken with sea salt and white pepper. Brown the chicken pieces, in small batches, on all sides in the hot oil. Remove as they are browned and set aside. Add extra olive oil as needed.

Once all the chicken is browned, use the same pan and oil to sauté the garlic, ginger, and chile on medium heat for 2 minutes. Add the cayenne, coriander, and turmeric and sauté for about 2 minutes, until the spices are well combined and release their fragrance. Add the cilantro and fry in the spiced oil for about 2 minutes. Once the herbs and spices are fried, remove about half the herbs with a slotted spoon and set aside. Place the chicken back into the pan. Add the lemon juice and water and bring to a boil over high heat. Once boiling, turn the heat to low, cover, and cook for 15 minutes. Turn the chicken pieces over and cook another 15 minutes, until tender.

Serve the chicken pieces over a bed of basmati rice. Spoon the accumulated sauce over the chicken and rice. Top with the reserved crispy cilantro.

BUTTERFLIED ROSEMARY CHICKEN WITH PAN JUICES

Protein, Vegetables, Healthy Fats
Detox, Level 1, Level 2

Serves 4

When Alan and I traveled to Tuscany to celebrate his seventieth birthday, an Italian housewife taught me to make this incredible chicken. It has all the flavor of a whole roasted chicken, but without the bones. You must make friends with your butcher to make this dish a reality. The first time I asked my butcher to remove all the bones from my organic roasting chicken, it took him a very long time! Now I know to call in advance and order it. I always ask for the bones in a separate package so I can make incredible homemade broth.

One 5-pound roasting chicken, deboned and butterflied
4 tablespoons olive oil
1 tablespoon turmeric
Sea salt and freshly ground black pepper
1 bunch fresh rosemary
4 tablespoons (½ stick) unsalted butter
1 cup chicken broth, preferably homemade (see page 260)

Preheat the oven to 350 degrees.

Lay the chicken skin side up in a roasting pan. Make a paste with the olive oil and the turmeric and brush it liberally over the entire chicken, then season with sea salt and pepper. Lay twigs of fresh rosemary on top of the chicken and dot with half of the butter. Place the roasting pan in the oven and cook for about 1 hour. The skin should be crispy. If it is not crispy, turn on the broiler and crisp the skin under it for a couple of minutes. Keep an eye on it, as it can burn quickly.

To make a light sauce from the pan drippings, remove the chicken and herbs from the pan and place onto a cutting board. Pour most of the fat out of the roasting pan, reserving about 1 tablespoon. Place the pan onto the stovetop, turn the heat to high, and add the chicken broth, scraping the browned bits from the bottom. Boil until the liquid is reduced by half. Turn off the heat, then add the remaining butter and swirl until combined and smooth.

Carve the chicken. Spoon the buttery juices onto each plate, and lay the chicken pieces on top with a sprinkle of the crispy rosemary.

SOUTHWEST ROASTED CHICKEN

Protein, Healthy Fats
Detox, Level 1, Level 2

Serves 4

Like many households, we eat a lot of chicken. I usually default to my typical Italian/Tuscan seasonings, but one day I decided to spice it up with my Southwest Sea Salt Rub, which makes for a very easy, delicious dinner. Since Alan doesn't eat any gluten, I made Asparagus Jalapeño Risotto (page 244) to go with it. Great dinner for Level 2—and nice to have a little variety! This chicken on its own is good for Detox and Level 1.

  One 4- to 5-pound organic whole chicken
  Extra virgin olive oil
  1 to 2 tablespoons SUZANNE Southwest Sea Salt Rub (See Note)
  2 cups chicken broth

Preheat the oven to 350 degrees.

Remove the giblets from the chicken and set aside. Rinse the chicken and pat dry. Place it into a roasting pan with the giblets. Drizzle olive oil over the entire chicken. Rub the chicken all over with Suzanne Southwest Sea Salt Rub or your own blend.

Roast for about 1 hour and 20 minutes (about 20 minutes per pound). Remove the chicken from the pan. Place the roasting pan onto the stovetop over medium-high heat. Add the chicken broth and boil, scraping the browned bits from the bottom of the pan, until the pan drippings are syrupy. Serve the sliced chicken with a spoonful of the sauce.

Note: You can also make your own spice blend. Combine 2 cloves garlic, minced, 1 tablespoon sea salt, 1 teaspoon cumin seeds, 1 teaspoon ancho chili powder, ½ teaspoon oregano, ½ teaspoon sage, and ¼ teaspoon thyme.

🌿 CHICKEN PATTY PICCATA 🌿

Protein, Vegetables, Healthy Fats
Detox, Level 1, Level 2

Serves 4

This is an easy and inexpensive way to make chicken piccata, using ground chicken. I prefer the dark ground chicken because the white tends to dry out too quickly.

2 pounds ground chicken
4 tablespoons extra virgin olive oil
½ cup chicken broth (see page 260)
Sea salt and freshly ground black pepper
1 tablespoon freshly chopped tarragon
3 tablespoons butter

Divide the ground chicken into 4 portions and shape them into patties about 1½ inches thick. Heat a sauté pan over high, add the olive oil, and fry the patties until cooked and crusty, about 2 to 3 minutes on each side. Remove the patties. Add the chicken broth to the skillet, scrape up all the bits from the bottom, and boil for about 3 minutes, or until the broth is reduced by half. Season with sea salt and pepper. Turn off the heat, add the chopped tarragon, then add the butter and slowly swirl it around until the butter smoothes out the sauce. Pour over the chicken patties and serve immediately.

MOZZARELLA-STUFFED
TURKEY BURGER

Protein, Vegetables, Healthy Fats
Detox, Level 1, Level 2

Serves 6

I love ground meat. When I come home from work and haven't thought about dinner until that time, if I have fresh ground meat in the refrigerator I know I can make something in minutes. Turkey can get dry—that's why I use dark turkey meat and add the mozzarella stuffed in the center, which keeps it moist and yummy. Serve with steamed broccoli for an easy, delicious meal.

2 pounds dark ground turkey
Sea salt and freshly ground black pepper
½ cup chopped fresh basil
6 ounces fresh mozzarella cheese, chopped into 1-inch chunks
3 tablespoons extra virgin olive oil

In a bowl, combine the turkey, sea salt, pepper, and basil. Form into 6 patties about 1½ inches thick. Stuff a few chunks of cheese into the center of the patties (about 3 chunks per patty). Heat a large sauté pan over medium high heat. Add the olive oil, then the patties in a single layer. Cook for 2 to 3 minutes on each side. Serve immediately.

🌿 CHICKEN BROTH 🌿

Protein, Vegetables, Healthy Fats
Detox, Level 1, Level 2

Makes approximately 10 cups

You can't have great soup if you don't start with a tasty broth. I have cre-ated several variations of broth over the years. This version comes from my housekeeper, Shirani. When I make my Butterflied Rosemary Chicken, I ask the butcher to debone the chicken, but I always get those bones in a sepa-rate bag to make stock! Shirani cooked the raw bones with the vegetables to make this wonderful broth. You may use a number of different vegetables or trimmings from vegetables. Throughout the week, gather any leftover veg-etables or trimmed pieces (in a sealable bag), such as stems of mushrooms, leftover celery, stems from herbs, etc. Store this bag in the freezer, and when you are ready to make stock, dump it into your soup pot. I also keep extra chicken carcasses in this bag, and since we eat a lot of chicken, I end up with very rich broth! I have included carrots, parsnips, and a corn cob in this recipe, but those would be allowed only for Level 2.

¼ cup olive oil
3 onions, coarsely chopped
4 to 6 leeks, quartered
Raw chicken bones
4 quarts water
6 stalks celery, quartered
15 mushrooms, cut in half
5 parsnips, cut in half
Stems from parsley
Any leftover trimmed vegetables, from the freezer
5 carrots, quartered (for Level 2)

1 corn husk (for Level 2)

Sea salt and freshly ground black pepper, to taste

Place a large stock pot over high heat. Add the olive oil, onions, and leeks. Sweat them to soften and create some brown bits on the bottom of the pot. Add the chicken bones and brown slightly, then add the water and the rest of the vegetables. Cook at a low boil for about 3 hours. Strain the stock into a colander with another pot underneath to catch the golden broth. Mash the vegetables against the colander to squeeze out all their good juices. Discard the vegetables and bones. Store the stock in 1-quart containers in the freezer. Season with sea salt and pepper before using.

🌿 INDIAN-STYLE PETRALE SOLE 🌿

Protein, Vegetables, Healthy Fats
Detox, Level 1, Level 2

Serves 4

Petrale sole is a mild white fish—always one of my favorites. In this extremely quick and easy preparation, it's seasoned with the flavors of India for an earthy, delicious alternative to the traditional butter and lemon. (And so good for you, with these life-giving spices!) Serve with a steamed vegetable for a wonderful meal that won't keep you in the kitchen all night.

> 2 teaspoons ground cumin
> 1½ teaspoons turmeric
> 1 teaspoon cayenne
> 2 pounds fresh petrale sole (or other white fish)
> Sea salt and freshly ground black pepper
> ¼ cup finely chopped flat-leaf parsley
> Extra virgin olive oil
> Lemon wedges

Combine the cumin, turmeric, and cayenne in a small bowl. Set aside.

Season the fish all over with sea salt and black pepper. Distribute the blended spices evenly on both sides of the fish. Sprinkle the chopped parsley over fish, patting to make sure it adheres.

Place a large sauté pan over medium-high heat. Coat the bottom of the pan with olive oil. When the oil is hot, add the fish in a single layer, and fry about 3 minutes. Carefully flip and cook the other side for another 3 minutes. Serve with lemon wedges.

SEARED SALMON WITH
BASIL PARSLEY PESTO

Protein, Vegetables, Healthy Fats, Carbohydrates
Detox, Level 1, Level 2

Serves 2

Salmon—it's pink, beautiful, and full of healthy omega-3 fats. Even though I am not a huge fish eater, I had to give you a simple recipe for this amazing superfood. Apply the small amount of carbohydrates from the pine nuts in the pesto to your daily guidelines.

Two 6-ounce fillets wild-caught salmon
Sea salt and freshly ground black pepper
3 tablespoons extra virgin olive oil
4 tablespoons Basil Parsley Pesto (page 221)
Lemon wedges

Preheat the oven to 350 degrees.

Season the salmon with sea salt and pepper. Place an oven-safe pan over medium-high heat. Add the olive oil and the salmon and sear for 2 to 3 minutes on each side to create a crusty coating. Place the entire pan in the oven and roast for 5 minutes, until the center is just cooked through. Carefully remove from the heat (the handle will be hot) and place the fish on a serving dish. Top each fillet with a generous dollop of pesto and serve with a lemon wedge.

PORK CHOPS
🌿 IN CREAMY MUSHROOM 🌿
TARRAGON SAUCE

Protein, Vegetables, Healthy Fats
Detox, Level 1, Level 2

Serves 4

I love pan-fried pork chops. They take on a crusty, savory taste from the sea salt and the olive oil. What's left in the bottom of the frypan is the most delicious part. From this I can make the most incredible sauces. Shiitake mushrooms are loaded with antioxidants, as is the fresh tarragon. Pork is great protein, and you are getting a detoxifying effect along with your protein for this meal.

> 4 center-cut pork chops, 1½ inches thick, on the bone
> Sea salt and freshly ground black pepper
> ¼ cup freshly chopped tarragon leaves
> 6 tablespoons olive oil
> ¼ pound (about 10) shiitake mushrooms, sliced
> ½ cup chicken broth (see page 260)
> ¼ cup heavy cream

Season the pork chops with sea salt and pepper and half of the tarragon.

Heat a large frypan on high and add 3 tablespoons of the olive oil. Add the pork chops in a single layer and cook 3 to 4 minutes on each side. Remove from the pan and set aside to keep warm. Add the remaining oil, then the sliced mushrooms, and sauté on high heat, 5 to 7 minutes, until crusty. Add the chicken broth and scrape the bits from the bottom of the pan to release the flavor. Reduce the broth by half, then add the cream and the rest of the fresh tarragon. (If the sauce is too thick, add a little more chicken broth.) Adjust the seasonings as needed. Cook for 1 to 2 minutes, until the sauce is bubbling. Spoon over the pork chops and serve immediately.

🌿 SPICY PORK CHOPS 🌿

··

Protein, Vegetables, Healthy Fats
Level 1, Level 2

Serves 4

Pork chops are a crowd-pleaser. The white meat is sweet and tender and absorbs flavor beautifully. If you can find organic pork, it is so much healthier and tastier. Because of the white wine, we save this for Level 2.

    ¼ cup whole-grain mustard
    6 cloves garlic, minced
    1 cup white wine (omit for Level 1)
    ¼ cup agave nectar
    6 shoulder pork chops, about 1½ inches thick
    Extra virgin olive oil
    Sea salt and freshly ground black pepper

In a small glass bowl, make a marinade with the mustard, garlic, white wine, and agave. Place the pork chops into the marinade and set aside for about 15 minutes, in the refrigerator.

Heat a large sauté pan on medium high. When hot, add the olive oil, then pull the pork chops out of the marinade and place them into the hot pan in a single layer. Sauté about 3 to 4 minutes on each side. Remove from pan, season with sea salt and pepper, and serve immediately.

✄ LAMB CARNITAS ✄

....

Protein, Vegetables, Healthy Fats
Detox, Level 1, Level 2

Serves 8

My Mother's Day lunch this year was as delicious as ever! It's typically my favorite day of the year; and this was no exception. Bruce and my granddaughters set the table outside with white French plates and garden roses, while Caroline was busy in the kitchen creating a twist on an old favorite recipe. The inspiration started with a sale on organic New Zealand lamb shoulder. We always try to eat grass-fed meat, and when good local organic isn't around, we eat New Zealand meat as it's known for its good quality. Caroline makes incredible carnitas with pork shoulder, so she decided to try it with lamb . . . and the result was fantastic! We ate these crispy little salted pieces of lamb served in a cabbage leaf cup with Mikri Greek Salad (page 219), and Hummus on Fire (page 220)—and whole-wheat pita for those who wished to partake. I am one lucky mother!

    4 pounds lamb shoulder, cut into 2-inch cubes
    2 teaspoons sea salt
    1 head purple or green cabbage
    Olive oil, if needed

Place the lamb cubes into a large sauté pan or heavy-bottomed Dutch oven. Season generously with sea salt. Fill the pan with water so that it barely covers the meat and turn the heat to high. Bring to a boil, then lower the heat to medium and let the meat continue to cook until all the liquid has evaporated. By this time the meat will be cooked through but not yet falling apart. Allow the meat to continue cooking until all the fat has been rendered out. Now the lamb will begin to brown in its own juices. Be careful to scrape the bottom of the pan consistently to create the crispiness, and to keep the carnitas from burning. The lamb is done when it's crispy on the edges and starts shredding into pieces. Allow 60 to 80 minutes for the complete cooking process. Toward the end of the cooking process, feel free to add a little olive oil if your pieces are not crispy enough.

Spoon carnitas into a cabbage leaf and serve with Mikri Greek Salad and Hummus on Fire.

MIDDLE EASTERN
LAMB CHOPS

Protein, Vegetables, Healthy Fats, Carbohydrates
Level 1, Level 2

Serves 2

Cardamom is a spice few of us understand how to use, but it gives an interesting new twist to lamb. Shoulder cuts are best and cheapest; just don't burn them. Count the small amount of yogurt toward your Carbohydrates.

½ cup whole-milk yogurt, preferably Greek
2 lemons
¼ teaspoon cardamom
½ cup fresh mint, roughly chopped
4 shoulder lamb chops
Extra virgin olive oil
Sea salt and freshly ground black pepper
Parsley sprigs, for garnish

In a medium-size mixing bowl, combine the yogurt with the juice of 1 lemon, the cardamom, and mint. Marinate the lamb chops in this mixture for about 10 minutes. Heat a skillet on high. Add olive oil, then pull the chops from the marinade and fry in the pan for 2 to 3 minutes on each side. Season with sea salt and pepper and serve with a lemon wedge and sprigs of parsley.

🌿 LAMB BURGER, GREEK STYLE 🌿

Protein, Vegetables, Healthy Fats, Carbohydrates
Detox, Level 1, Level 2

Serves 6

Here's a great twist on the traditional hamburger—it's a lamb burger, topped with all the things I love about Greek food: feta, tomato, olives, red onion, and oregano. And since we don't need that yucky white flour, we've left off the bun. You will not miss it. Count the olives toward your Carbohydrates, and omit them for Detox.

> 2 pounds ground lamb
> Sea salt and freshly ground black pepper
> 1 tablespoon dried oregano
> 4 tablespoons extra virgin olive oil
> 6 ounces feta cheese, grated
> 2 ripe tomatoes, sliced
> ½ red onion, thinly sliced
> ½ cup chopped Kalamata olives (omit for Detox)
> 2 Persian cucumbers, chopped

Place the lamb in a bowl. Season well with sea salt, pepper, and oregano. Mash together with your hands to combine. Shape the seasoned meat into 6 patties about 1½ inches thick.

In a sauté pan set over medium-high heat add the olive oil, then the patties in a single layer. Cook for 2 to 3 minutes on each side. Remove from the heat.

Sprinkle immediately with the grated feta so it melts a little. Top with sliced tomato, a slice of red onion, a spoonful of olives, and a spoonful of cucumbers. Serve immediately.

🌿 BLUE CHEESE BURGERS 🌿

Protein, Vegetables, Healthy Fats, Carbohydrates, Fruit
Level 2

Serves 6

I love a great salad with arugula, blue cheese, toasted walnuts, and fresh pear slices. One day I was serving this salad and also testing some delicious natural burgers from an organic farmer in Nevada. The combo inspired this burger! It's another easy, inexpensive meal with ground meat, but gourmet and delicious. This is Level 2 because of the pear. If you left off the fruit, you could eat it during Level 1, with the nuts counting toward your Carbohydrates.

2 pounds ground beef
1 cup crumbled blue cheese
½ cup chopped toasted walnuts
Sea salt and freshly ground black pepper
4 tablespoons olive oil
1 pear, cored and sliced (omit for Level 1)
2 bunches arugula

In a mixing bowl, combine the ground beef, blue cheese, walnuts, sea salt, and pepper. Divide the meat into 6 portions and shape into patties about 1½ inches thick.

Heat a large skillet on high. When hot, add the olive oil, then the patties in a single layer. Cook for 2 to 3 minutes on each side. Remove the burgers. Add a little more olive oil to the pan, then add the pear slices. Fry until soft.

Place each burger on a bed of fresh arugula lightly drizzled with olive oil and sea salt, top with some sliced pears, and serve immediately.

BEEF TENDERLOIN MEDALLIONS

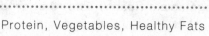

Protein, Vegetables, Healthy Fats
Detox, Level 1, Level 2

Serves 2

This recipe uses one of the most tender cuts of beef; I guess that's why it's called the *tender*loin! I always ask my butcher for grass-fed beef, cut into ¼-inch slices, and pounded lightly, as you would for Veal or Chicken Piccata. The thin slices only need to be cooked for a minute or two on each side, so they retain their juices and flavor. I like to rub a smashed clove of garlic on both sides, sprinkle with olive oil, and add a sprig or two of fresh rosemary, then let sit in the refrigerator until guests arrive or it's dinnertime for the family. This is simple to prepare, yet a very elegant and sumptuous offering. I serve with roasted tomatoes, which interact with the goat cheese beautifully, and salad greens.

8 ounces beef tenderloin, sliced and pounded to ¼ inch thick
4 garlic cloves, smashed
4 tablespoons extra virgin olive oil
Sea salt and freshly ground black pepper
4 sprigs fresh rosemary
½ pound baby greens
1 fresh lemon
6 ounces goat cheese, cut into 8 slices

Place the beef medallions on a large platter. Rub with the smashed garlic, brush with 2 tablespoons of the olive oil, then season with sea salt and pepper and lay the rosemary sprigs on top. Set aside, or refrigerate until ready to cook.

Prepare the salad greens by drizzling with a little olive oil, sea salt, pepper, and a squeeze of fresh lemon.

Heat a large sauté pan on medium high. Add the remaining 2 tablespoons olive oil, then the medallions in a single layer, and sauté for 1 to 2 minutes on each side. Return the cooked meat to a serving platter and top each slice with a little goat cheese and the dressed baby greens. Serve immediately.

Desserts

CHOCOLATE PEANUT BUTTER SQUARES

Healthy Fats, Carbohydrates, Insulin Triggers
Level 2

Serves 12

I fell in love with this dessert at an Asian restaurant. I was able to sweet-talk the pastry chef into giving me the ingredient list. These squares are a good option for Level 2 since they contain no flour, and they are sinfully good! Just don't talk yourself into more than one!

    10 ounces dark chocolate (60% cocoa), coarsely chopped
    ½ cup creamy peanut butter, room temperature
    ¾ cup whole milk
    ¼ teaspoon sea salt
    1 cup heavy cream
    ½ cup chopped toasted peanuts
    Shaved chocolate pieces, for garnish

Butter a 9-by-9-inch pan.

Melt the chocolate in the top of a double boiler or in a heatproof bowl over a pan of simmering water. Stir occasionally until the chocolate has melted and is smooth. Remove from the heat. Transfer the melted chocolate to the bowl of a stand mixer. Add the peanut butter and briefly set aside.

In a small saucepan, bring the milk and salt to a boil. Add half of the milk to the peanut butter mixture and blend on low until incorporated, then add the remaining milk and blend until smooth. Increase the speed to high and whip for 5 minutes, or until the mixture is creamy and cooled to room temperature.

(continued)

In a clean bowl, whip the cream just until soft mounds form. Do not over-whip. Fold the cream into the peanut butter mixture. Spread the batter evenly into the prepared pan, cover, and let set in the refrigerator for at least 4 hours.

To serve, run a knife along the edge of the pan to loosen the sides and cut into squares. Place the squares onto serving plates and garnish with chopped peanuts and shaved chocolate pieces. It's best to soften these for about 10 minutes before serving.

PEPITA AND CACAO
NIB BRITTLE

Healthy Fats, Carbohydrates
Level 1, Level 2

Makes 1½ cups

This is a great treat and made with good carbohydrates. You may have small amounts of this on Level 1, counting toward your Carbohydrates. This yummy chewy brittle helps keep you away from the sugary treats. Cacao is the unsweetened nib used to make chocolate. It's available in most specialty shops and some grocery stores. It's worth the hunt because when you want a treat, you will love having this brittle to nibble on to satiate that craving. There is quite a bit of SomerSweet in the recipe, so watch out for the fiber effect!

¼ cup unsweetened cacao nibs
¾ cup raw pepitas (pumpkin seeds)
½ cup All Natural SomerSweet
¼ cup water
⅛ teaspoon cream of tartar
Pinch of cayenne pepper (optional)

Coarsely chop the cacao nibs and transfer them to a small strainer. Save the powdery pieces for another dessert. Use the slightly larger pieces to make a clearer brittle.

Toast the pumpkin seeds in a small skillet over medium heat, shaking often, until they begin to pop, 5 to 7 minutes. Remove the seeds from heat and set aside.

Line a baking sheet with parchment paper and grease the parchment with a little butter.

(continued)

In a medium saucepan, combine the sweetener, water, and cream of tartar. Bring to a simmer over medium heat, stirring until the sweetener dissolves. Lower the heat to medium-low, cover, and let simmer for 2 to 3 minutes. Remove the pan lid and brush crystals from the sides of the pan with a wet pastry brush. Continue simmering for 3 to 5 minutes, or until the syrup begins to color. Watch closely because the caramel can burn quickly. Test the color of the caramel by drizzling a few drops on a white plate. When the color is medium to dark amber, remove the pan from the heat and stir in the nibs, pepitas, and optional cayenne.

Working quickly, pour the mixture into the prepared pan and spread it as thinly as possible with a heatproof spatula or wooden spoon.

Allow the brittle to cool completely, then break it into small pieces. Store in an airtight container for up to 4 days.

FLOURLESS CHOCOLATE PECAN CAKES

Carbohydrates, Healthy Fats, Insulin Triggers
Level 2

Makes 12

These delicious individual cakes are made with ground pecans instead of flour. For you chocolate lovers, a great Level 2 dessert!

8 ounces dark chocolate (at least 60% cocoa)
6 ounces unsalted butter
1¼ cups All Natural SomerSweet
¾ cup finely ground pecans
1 cup cocoa powder, sifted
5 eggs
Whipped cream, for serving (optional)

Preheat the oven to 325 degrees. Grease twelve 4-ounce heatproof custard cups (or muffin tins).

Place the chocolate, butter, and sweetener into the top of a double boiler or in a heatproof bowl over a pan of simmering water. Stir until melted.

In a separate bowl, combine the ground pecans and cocoa powder. Add the melted chocolate and whisk together. Add the eggs, one at a time, whisking until combined.

Spoon the batter into the cups or tins. Bake for 25 minutes, until a toothpick inserted into the center comes out just slightly moist. Remove from the oven, and cool in the cups for at least 15 minutes. Invert onto dessert plates and serve with whipped cream, if desired.

✌ CHOCOLATE MOUSSE ✌

Protein, Healthy Fats, Carbohydrates, Insulin Triggers
Level 2

Serves 6

Yummy, soft, chocolatey, and very low in sugar! You will never know the difference between this and a sugary dessert. This is just what chocolate mousse should be. For a Level 1 option, try my SUZANNE Chocolate Mousse Mix.

12 ounces dark chocolate (at least 60% cocoa), finely chopped
4 large egg yolks
1 cup whole milk
4 tablespoons All Natural SomerSweet (or sugar)
⅔ cup heavy cream
Chocolate shavings, for garnish

Place the chocolate in a large bowl, with a fine-mesh strainer over the bowl.

In a medium bowl, stir together the egg yolks. In a medium saucepan, bring the milk and 2 tablespoons of the sweetener to a simmer, stirring until it has dissolved. Slowly pour the milk into the eggs, stirring constantly with a heatproof rubber spatula or wooden spoon. Pour the mixture back into the saucepan and cook, stirring constantly, over medium heat for 6 to 10 minutes, until the mixture is thick enough to coat the back of a wooden spoon. Remove from the heat and strain the custard into the chocolate. Stir gently until the chocolate has melted completely. Let cool to room temperature.

In a chilled bowl, whip the cream until it holds soft peaks, and whip in the remaining sweetener until the cream holds its shape. Do not overwhip or the mousse will get grainy.

Fold together the whipped cream and the chocolate mixture. (Reserve a little whipped cream for serving.) Cover with plastic wrap and refrigerate for at least 4 hours.

To serve, place a dollop of whipped cream on the bottom of each dessert dish (I like to use martini glasses) and scoop the mousse on top of the cream. Garnish with a sprinkle of shaved chocolate.

🌿 COCOA NUTS 🌿

Protein, Carbohydrates, Healthy Fats
Level 1, Level 2

Makes about 6 cups

I'm always looking for tasty, low-sugar desserts. These nuts are coated with a soft meringue and then baked. The result is a satisfying crispy combo of nuts and sweet meringues. Keep these on hand for something sweet in Level 1, but remember not to overdo it, and count them toward your Carbohydrates.

> 2 cups pecan halves
> 1 cup walnut halves
> 6 tablespoons unsalted butter, cut into cubes
> 2 large egg whites
> 1 cup All Natural SomerSweet
> 1 tablespoon unsweetened cocoa powder

Preheat the oven to 325 degrees.

Spread the nuts on a baking sheet and toast for 10 minutes. Remove the nuts from the baking sheet and set aside. Scatter the butter pieces over the baking sheet and place in the oven to melt. Remove from oven as soon as the butter is melted.

With an electric mixer, whip the egg whites until they just start to hold a shape. With the mixer running, gradually add the sweetener, and continue to whip for 2 minutes. The mixture will be sticky and shiny, much thinner than a typical meringue. Sift the cocoa on top of the whites and fold in the nuts with a spatula.

Scoop the nut-meringue mixture onto the buttered baking sheet and gently spread it out. Bake for 10 minutes. Remove the pan from the oven and use a metal spatula to break up the nut mixture and turn the pieces in the butter. Return to the oven for another 10 minutes, then break up the nuts and turn them again. Return to the oven for a final 15 minutes. When done, the butter will be mostly absorbed, the coating will be dry, and the nuts will be robed in a crispy meringue. Place the pan on a cooling rack and let cool completely.

Break up clumps and store in an airtight container for up to a week.

🌿 NUTTY CHOCOLATE TORTE 🌿

Protein, Healthy Fats, Carbohydrates, Insulin Triggers
Level 2

Serves 12

Chocoholic alert! This dark, dense chocolate cake is so rich and delicious you
only need a small slice. Use a very good-quality dark chocolate, like Valrhona
or Scharffenberger. (If you can find a good sugar-free chocolate, you may use
it.) If I have time, I like to toast the nuts before I grind them in the food processor. This cake is lower in flour and sugar than a regular chocolate cake—and
sinfully delicious.

16 ounces dark chocolate (at least 60% cocoa)
1 cup unsalted butter
1 cup ground nuts (hazelnuts, almonds, pecans, or walnuts)
½ cup whole-wheat pastry flour
7 eggs, separated
1 cup All Natural SomerSweet (or sugar)
½ cup brandy
Whipped cream, for serving

Preheat the oven to 325 degrees. Butter and flour a 10-inch cake pan, preferably a springform pan.

Melt the chocolate and butter in the top of a double boiler, or in a heatproof bowl over a saucepan of simmering water. Set aside to cool.

Combine the ground nuts and flour in a bowl and set aside.

Beat the egg yolks until light and fluffy. Slowly add the sweetener and
continue beating until the mixture is pale yellow and tripled in volume.

Fold in the melted chocolate. Fold in the flour mixture. Then fold in the brandy.

In a separate bowl, beat the egg whites until soft peaks form. Gently fold them into the batter in two batches. Spread the batter evenly in the prepared pan and tap on the counter to eliminate air pockets. Bake for about 45 minutes, or until a toothpick inserted into the center comes out slightly moist.

Set aside to cool on a rack for at least 1 hour. Since the center may be moist, it's best to refrigerate it for 2 hours. Release the sides of pan and invert cake. Slice and serve with whipped cream.

🌿 RASPBERRY CRÈME BRÛLÉE 🌿

Protein, Healthy Fats, Fruit
Level 1, Level 2

Serves 8

Crème Brûlée is a decadent, rich custard with a thin layer of caramelized sugar on top. And since it's mostly fats, it creates less of an insulin response. This recipe is a great option that can keep you away from sugary desserts. If you are going to enjoy this on Level 1, make sure you do not have any carbohydrates with it! The slight imbalance from the berries is no problem, as long as you are steadily losing on Level 1. If you make it with sugar, only enjoy it on Level 2.

> 1 pint fresh raspberries
> 1½ cups heavy cream
> 1 vanilla bean, split lengthwise
> 9 large egg yolks
> ⅓ cup plus 8 tablespoons All Natural SomerSweet (or sugar)
> Mint leaves, for garnish

Lightly butter eight 5-inch heatproof ramekins or individual soufflé dishes. Place a few raspberries into the bottom of each dish. Fill a large bowl with ice cubes. Set aside.

In a medium saucepan, combine the heavy cream with the vanilla bean and its scrapings. Bring to a boil over low heat.

Place the egg yolks and the ⅓ cup sweetener into the top of a double boiler, or in a heatproof bowl over a pan of simmering water. Whisk vigorously until the mixture becomes a very pale yellow and feels hot to the touch. Remove from the heat and whisk in the boiling cream. Place back on the pan of simmering water, but turn off the heat. Whisk the mixture until it thickens, 5 to 10 minutes.

When the mixture has thickened, place the top of the double boiler into the larger bowl filled with the ice cubes. Whisk occasionally to cool. Strain into a clean bowl.

Spoon the custard into the prepared ramekins and refrigerate, covered, until firm, about 2 hours. When ready to serve, sprinkle 1 tablespoon of All Natural SomerSweet evenly over the top of each serving. Caramelize with a propane torch, or set 1 inch from a hot broiler until the tops brown. Garnish with more raspberries and mint leaves.

NEW YORK–STYLE
🌿 CHEESECAKE WITH 🌿
LEMON ESSENCE

Protein, Healthy Fats
Detox, Level 1, Level 2

Serves 8

This rich, delicious cheesecake is made from eggs, full-fat cream cheese, and real sour cream. A small slice is enough to make you feel wonderfully indulged, and if you make it with my All Natural SomerSweet, it won't spike your insulin. Still, maintain control! Small amounts during the Detox Phase, then you may start enjoying it, in moderation, on Level 1 when you are losing steadily. If you make it with sugar, only enjoy it on Level 2.

Two 8-ounce packages cream cheese
½ cup All Natural SomerSweet (or sugar)
3 large eggs
Zest of 1 lemon
4 tablespoons fresh lemon juice
2 teaspoons vanilla extract
¼ teaspoon salt
3 cups sour cream
Lemon slices, for garnish

Preheat the oven to 350 degrees. In a large mixing bowl, beat the cream cheese and sweetener until very smooth, about 3 minutes. Add the eggs, one at a time, beating well after each addition. Add the lemon zest, lemon juice, vanilla, and salt. Beat in the sour cream until just blended.

Grease an 8-inch springform pan with 2½-inch sides and line the bottom with greased parchment paper. Wrap the outside of the pan with a double layer of heavy-duty foil to prevent seepage.

Pour the batter into the pan. Set the pan in a large roasting pan and surround with 1 inch of very hot water. Bake for 45 minutes. Turn off the oven without opening the door and let the cake sit in the oven for 1 hour. Remove to a rack and cool to room temperature, about 1 hour. Cover with plastic wrap and refrigerate overnight. Unmold the cake onto a serving plate and garnish with lemon slices.

🌿 BERRY COMPOTE 🌿

Fruit, Insulin Triggers
Level 2

Serves 8

Berry Compote could also be called the world's easiest berry pie—because there's no crust! It's like having all of that gooey berry pie filling with none of the hassle of making dough, chilling it, and rolling it out. Just toss those fresh berries together with a couple of ingredients and bake. Wonderful with a little whipped cream or vanilla ice cream. The cornstarch thickens the compote, but you could try it without that ingredient if you'd like to enjoy this treat on Detox or Level 1. It will be runnier but still delicious.

   8 cups frozen or fresh berries (blueberries, blackberries, raspberries,
      strawberries)
   2 tablespoons cornstarch
   ½ cup orange juice
   ¾ cup All Natural SomerSweet
   Ice cream or whipped cream, for serving

Preheat the oven to 425 degrees.

Place the berries into a large bowl. In a small bowl, combine the cornstarch and orange juice. Stir until well combined. Add sweetener and stir to combine. Pour the mixture over berries. Gently stir to coat all the berries.

Pour the berries into a 9-by-9-inch baking dish. Bake for 15 minutes, then reduce the heat to 350 degrees and bake for 30 minutes more, until the juices are thick and bubbly. Remove from the oven. Spoon into bowls and top each serving with a scoop of high-quality vanilla ice cream or whipped cream.

FOOD REFERENCE GUIDE

Here are complete lists of foods for each of the categories within the plan. As always, organic is best, when available and affordable. First up: the foods and food ingredients to avoid as you get started on this new way of eating. For printable versions of these lists, and access to a Sexy Forever nutrition coach, join SexyForever.com/book.

- Detox: Eliminate all Insulin Triggers.

- Level 1—Weight Loss: Eliminate all Insulin Triggers, except for extremely rare occasions when you have no other choices. Then get right back on track.

- Level 2—Lifestyle: Eat Insulin Triggers in moderation only.

FOODS AND FOOD INGREDIENTS TO AVOID

INSULIN TRIGGERS

Sugars

Brown sugar	Molasses
Corn syrup	Raw sugar
High-fructose corn syrup	Sucrose
Honey	White sugar
Maple syrup	

Starchy Fruits and Vegetables

Acorn squash	Hubbard squash
Beets	Parsnips
Bananas	Potatoes
Butternut squash	Pumpkin
Carrots	Sweet potatoes
Corn	Yams

Refined Grains

White flour	White rice
White pasta	

Alcohol

Beer	Wine
Hard alcohol	

Caffeine

Caffeinated coffee or tea (Note: 1 cup coffee or tea is allowed per day, without other food)	Caffeinated sodas

---

BAD FATS

Trans Fats

The most dangerous of all fats—eliminate completely.

Margarine or spreads made with partially hyrogenated oils	Partially hydrogenated oils
	Shortening made with partially hyrogenated oils

Omega-6 Oils

While it is virtually impossible to eliminate them, reduce your intake as much as possible.

Corn

Cottonseed

Peanut

Safflower

Soybean

Sunflower

Vegetable

CHEMICALS, ADDITIVES, ARTIFICIAL FLAVORS, ARTIFICIAL COLORS, PRESERVATIVES

This is a list of the ingredients in food you should try to avoid to reduce your toxic burden.

acetylated esters of mono- and diglycerides

ammonium chloride

artificial colors

artificial flavors

aspartame

azodicarbonamide

benzoates

benzoyl peroxide

BHA (butylated hydroxyanisole)

BHT (butylated hydroxytoluene)

bleached flour

bromated flour

brominated vegetable oil (BVO)

calcium bromate

calcium disodium EDTA

calcium peroxide

calcium propionate

calcium saccharin

calcium sorbate

calcium stearoyl-2-lactylate

caprocaprylobehenin

certified colors

cyclamates

cysteine (l-cysteine), as an additive for bread products

DATEM (diacetyl tartaric and fatty acid esters of mono- and diglycerides)

dimethylpolysiloxane

dioctyl sodium sulfosuccinate (DSS)

disodium calcium EDTA

disodium dihydrogen EDTA

disodium guanylate

disodium inosinate

ethyl vanillin

ethylene oxide

ethyoxyquin

FD&C colors

food in lead-soldered cans

GMP (disodium guanylate)

hexa-, hepta-, and octa-esters
   of sucrose

IMP (disodium inosinate)

irradiated foods

lactylated esters of mono- and
   diglycerides

methyl silicon

methylparaben

microparticularized whey-
   protein-derived fat
   substitute

monosodium glutamate
   (MSG)

natamycin

nitrates/nitrites

polydextrose

potassium benzoate

potassium bisulfite

potassium bromate

potassium metabisulfite

potassium sorbate

propionates

propyl gallate

propylparaben

saccharin

sodium aluminum phosphate

sodium aluminum sulfate

sodium benzoate

sodium bisulfite

sodium diacetate

sodium glutamate

sodium nitrate/nitrite

sodium propionate

sodium stearoyl-2-lactylate

sodium sulfite

solvent-extracted oils, as stand-
   alone single-ingredient oils
   (except grapeseed oil)

sorbic acid

sucralose

sucroglycerides

sucrose polyester

sulfites (sulfur dioxide)

TBHQ (tertiary
   butylhydroquinone)

tetrasodium EDTA

vanillin

FOODS TO EAT

PROTEIN

Eggs

I recommend organic, cage-free, DHA, omega-3 eggs. One serving equals 2 eggs.

Fish

Wild-caught is best. Avoid farmed fish. A reasonable serving equals 6 ounces. Try to rarely eat fish high in mercury, like tuna and swordfish.

Anchovies	Pollock
Bass	Pompano
Bluefish	Red snapper
Bonito	Sablefish
Burbot	Salmon
Carp	Sardines
Catfish	Sea bass
Cod	Shark
Eel	Smelt
Flatfish	Snapper
Flounder	Sole
Gefilte fish	Sturgeon
Grouper	Swordfish
Haddock	Tripe
Halibut	Trout
Herring	Tuna
Mackerel	Turbot
Mahimahi	Whitefish
Monkfish	Wolf fish
Ocean perch	Yellowtail
Orange roughy	

Other Seafood

A reasonable serving equals 6 ounces.

Abalone	Mussels
Caviar	Octopus
Clams	Oysters
Crab	Scallops
Crayfish	Shrimp
Lobster	Squid

Meat

Avoid corn-fed. Organic is best, then natural with no hormones or antibiotics. No nitrates or nitrites. A reasonable serving equals 6 ounces.

Bacon	Pastrami
Canadian bacon	Pepperoni
Beef	Pork
Bologna	Prosciutto
Bratwurst	Rabbit
Capicola	Salami
Cold cuts	Sausage
Ham	Veal
Hot dogs	Venison
Lamb	

Poultry

Organic, cage-free is best; next best is natural with no hormones or antibiotics. A reasonable serving equals 6 ounces.

Capon	Guinea fowl
Chicken	Pheasant
Cornish game hen	Quail
Duck	Squab
Goose	Turkey

HEALTHY FATS

Oils

Olive oil—this should be your
    staple; extra virgin is best
Grapeseed oil

Flaxseed oil
Mayonnaise—best made from
    light olive or grapeseed oils

Dairy Fats

Butter
Cream

Crème fraîche
Sour cream

Cheese

Asiago
Bel paese
Blue
Boursin
Brie
Buffalo mozzarella
Camembert
Cheddar
Colby
Cottage cheese (full fat)
Cream cheese
Farmer
Feta
Fontina
Goat
Gouda
Gruyère

Havarti
Hoop
Jarlsberg
Limburger
Mascarpone
Monterey jack
Mozzarella
Muenster
Parmesan
Pecorino Romano
Provolone
Queso blanco
Ricotta
Roquefort
String
Swiss

CARBOHYDRATES

Detox: Up to 3 servings per day
Level 1: Up to 4 servings per day
Level 2: At your discretion

Beans

A serving equals ½ cup cooked.

Adzuki	Kidney
Anasazi	Lentils
Black	Lima
Black-eyed peas	Mung
Cannellini	Navy
Fava	Pinto
Garbanzo	Red
Great northern	Split peas
Green peas	White

Whole-Grain Products

These include breads, bagels, crackers, hot cereals, cold cereals, or pasta made from these whole grains. A serving equals 1 slice of bread, ½ bagel, 1 rice cake, or ½ cup cereal, pasta, or rice.

Amaranth	Oat
Barley	Pumpernickel
Bran	Quinoa
Brown rice	Rye
Buckwheat	Spelt
Kamut	Whole wheat
Millet	Wild rice

Nonfat Dairy Products

A serving equals ½ cup.

Nonfat cottage cheese	Nonfat sour cream
Nonfat milk	Nonfat soy milk
Nonfat rice milk	Nonfat yogurt
Nonfat ricotta cheese	Whey protein

Carbohydrates with Healthy Fats

These foods are listed here because they contain a combination of Carbohydrates with Healthy Fats. You will treat them as Carbohydrates.

Avocados—½ avocado	Nuts—about 10
Cocoa—unsweetened, ¼ cup	Olives—about 10
Coconut—½ cup, fresh or dried, unsweetened	Soy—about ½ cup (organic only, no GMO)
Liver—2 ounces	
Low-fat and whole milk, cottage cheese, ricotta, yogurt—½ cup	

VEGETABLES AND HERBS

A serving of vegetables equals 1 cup raw or ½ cup cooked. Eat at least 6 servings per day.

Alfalfa sprouts	Cabbage
Artichoke	Cauliflower
Arugula	Celery
Asparagus	Chervil
Bamboo shoots	Chicory greens
Basil	Chives
Bean sprouts	Cilantro
Beet greens	Clover sprouts
Bok choy	Collard greens
Broccoli	Crookneck squash
Brussels sprouts	Cucumber

Daikon
Dandelion greens
Dill weed
Eggplant
Endive
Escarole
Fennel
Garlic
Ginger
Green beans
Horseradish
Jicama
Kale
Kohlrabi
Leeks
Lettuce
   Boston or Bibb
   Frisée
   Green leaf
   Iceberg
   Limestone
   Red oak
   Romaine
Mushrooms
Mustard greens
Okra
Onion
Parsley
Peppers
   Bell
   Cherry
   Chile
   Pepperoncini

Pickles (except sweet)
Purslane
Radicchio
Radish
Rhubarb
Rosemary
Sage
Salsify
Sauerkraut
Scallions
Shallots
Snow peas
Spinach
Sugar snap peas
Swiss chard
Tarragon
Thyme
Tomatillo
Tomato
Turnip
Turnip greens
Water chestnuts
Watercress
Wax beans
Yard-long beans
Yellow beans
Zucchini

FRUIT

A serving equals 1 medium-size piece of fruit, or about ½ cup. I recommend 2 to 3 servings per day. It's best not to eat fruit after dinner, except berries.

Apple
Apricot
Asian pear
Berries
    Acai
    Blackberry
    Blueberry
    Boysenberry
    Cranberry
    Currant
    Elderberry
    Gooseberry
    Maqui
    Mulberry
    Ollaberry
    Raspberry
    Strawberry
Cherimoya
Cherries
Crabapple
Fig
Grapefruit
Grapes
Guava
Kiwi
Kumquat
Lemon
Lime

Loquat
Lychee
Mandarin orange
Mango
Melons
    Cantaloupe
    Casaba
    Crenshaw
    Honeydew
    Orange fleshed
    Sharlyn
    Watermelon
Nectarine
Orange
Papaya
Passionfruit
Peach
Pear
Persimmon
Pineapple
Plum
Pomegranate
Prickly pear
Pomelo
Quince
Star fruit
Tamarind
Tangerine

SKIN CARE
INGREDIENTS TO AVOID

As you know now, it's not just what you eat that can increase your toxic burden. This is a partial list (yes, partial! Frightening, isn't it?) of the chemicals and toxins to avoid rubbing on your face or body. Look for clean products without these ingredients.

1,2 hexanediol
acetamide MEA
acrylates copolymer
AHAs
alcloxa
aldioxa
alkyl benzoate
alpha arbutin
alpha hydroxy acids
aluminum glycinate
aluminum hydroxide
aluminum oxide
aluminum powder
amino-guanidine
aminomethyl propanol
aminopropyl ascorbyl
    phosphate
ammonium alum
ammonium laureth sulfate
ammonium lauryl sulfate

ammonium polacrylate
AMP
artificial colors
avobenzone
babassuamidopropalkonium
    chloride
behenalkonium chloride
behenamidopropyl
    hydroxyethyl
dimonium chloride
behenoxy dimethicone
behentrimonium
    methosulfate
benzalkonium chloride
benzethonium chloride
benzophenone
benzyl PCA
betaine
BHA (butylated
    hydroxyanisole)

BHT (butylated hydroxytoluene)
bis diglyceryl polyacyladipate-2
bismuth oxychloride
boron nitride
bronopol
bumetrizole
butyl methoxydibenzoylmethane
butylene glycol
butylparaben
C 11-15 pareth 12
C 12-14 olefin Sulfonate
C 12-15 alkyl benzoate
C 12-15 alkyl lactate
C 12-15 alkyl octanoate
C 13-14 isoparaffin
capryl isostearate
carbomer
Carbowax (polyethylene glycol)
carmine
castor oil/IPDI copolymer
CDE (cocomide DEA)
ceramide 2, 3
ceresin
certified colors
ceteareth 2-100
ceteareth 5-20
cetearyl ethylhexanote
cetearyl isononanoate
cetearyl methicone
ceteth-20 phosphate
cetrimonium bromide
cetrimonium chloride
cetyl betaine
chlorphenesin
cocamide betaine
cocamide DEA
cocamide MEA
cocamide MIPA
cocamidopropyl PG-dimonium chloride
cocamidopropyl PG-dimonium chloride phosphate
cocamidopropylamine oxide
cochineal
coco betaine
coco phosphatidyl PG-dimonium chloride
cocoamphocarboxyglycinate
cocodimonium hydroxypropyl hydrolyzed rice protein
colloidal minerals
colloidal silver
copolymer
corn glycol
cyclomethicone
cyclopentasiloxane
cyclotetrasiloxane
diazolidinyl urea
dicaprylyl carbonate
dicaprylyl ether
dicetyldimonium chloride
diethanolamine (DEA)
dihydroxyacetone
diisopropyl dimerate
dimethicone copolyol

dimethicone crosspolymer-3

dimethyl capramide

dimethyl oxobenzo dioasilane

dimethyl phenyl 2-butanol

dimethylpolysiloxane

dioctyl sodium sulfosuccinate (DSS)

dipalmitoyl hydroxyproline

dipentaerythrityl

dipentaerythrityl hexahydroxystearate/ hexastearate/hexarosinate

dipolyhydroxystearate

dipropylene glycol

disodium EDTA

disodium laureth sulfosuccinate

disodium oleamido succinate

distearate 75

disteardimonium hectoride

DMDM hydantoin

EGMS

emu oil

ethoxydiglycol

ethoxydiglycol oleate

ethyl acetate

ethyl diglycol (polyethylene glycol)

ethyl methoxycinnamate

ethyl vanillin

ethylene glycol

FD&C colors

fragrance, synthetic

fullerenes

germaben

Germall

glycereth-26

glycereth-7 cocoate

glyceryl isostearate

glyceryl polyacrylate

hexadecanol

hexahydroxystearate/ hexastearate/hexarosinate

hexylene glycol

homosalate

human placental protein

hydroquinone

hydrotalcite

hydroxyethyl acrylate/sodium acryloyldimethyl taurate copolymer

hydroxyethyl soyamide

hydroxypropyl polysiloxane

imidazolidinyl urea

iodopropynyl butylcarbamate

IPDI

isoceteth-20

isocetyl isostearate

isohexadecane

isopentyldiol

isopropyl methylphenol

isopropyl myristate

isopropyl titanium triisostearate

kojic acid

lactamidopropyl trimonium chloride

lactic acid

lauramide MEA

laureth-7

laurethsulfosuccinate

lauryl amidopropyl betaine

lauryl glucoside betaine

magnesium aluminum silicate

magnesium myristate

MEA-containing ingredients

melanin

methoxycinnamate

methyl gluceth-10

methyl glyceth-20

methyl glycol

methyl propanediol

methyl soyate

methylchloroisothiazolinone

methylisothiazolinone

methylparaben

methylsilanol mannuronate

microcrystalline wax

mineral oil

myristic acid

myristyl alcohol

myristyl ether sulfate

myristyl lactate

myristyl myristate

nitrocellulose

nonoxynol 10

nylon-12

octinoxate

octisalate

octocrylene

octyl dodecyl neopentanoate

octyl methoxycinnamate

octyldecanol

octyldodecanol

olefin sulfonate

oleth 2-50

oleth-3-phosphate

oleyl betaine

oleyl oleate

oxybenzone

PABA (para-aminobenzoic acid

panthenyl ethyl ether

panthenyl triacetate

para-aminobenzoic acid
   (PABA)

parabens

paraphenylenediamine

Parsol

PCA-ethyl cocoyl arginate

pearl powder

PEG (polyethylene glycol)

PEG-6 caprylic/capric
   glycerides

PEG-7 glyceryl cocoate

PEG-10 sunflower glycerides

PEG-20, 100 stearate

PEG-35 (stearate) castor oil

PEG-40 hydrogenated castor
   oil

PEG-55 propylene glycol
   oleate

PEG-120 methyl glucose
   dioleate

PEG-150 distearate

PEG-150 pentaerythrityl
   tetrastearate

pentaerythrityl distearate

pentaerythrityl tetra-di-t-butyl
  hydroxyhydrocinnamate

pentaerythrityl tetrastearate

pentasodium pentetate

pentylene glycol

petrolatum

phenyl-butyl-nitrate

phenylbenzimidazole-5-
  sulfonic acid

phenyltrimethicone

phthalate

placental protein

polaxamer 335

polyacrylamide

polybutene

polyethylene glycol (PEG)

polyglyceryl-10 behenate/
  eicosadioate

polyglyceryl-2
  dipolyhydroxystearate

polyglyceryl-3 diisostearate

polyglyceryl-3 polyricinoleate

polyglyceryl-3 ricinoleate

polyglyceryl-4 isostearate

polyimide 1

polyisobutene

polypropylene glycol

polyquaternium 7, 10, 11

polysilicone-11, -15

polyvinylpyrrolidone

potassium alum

potassium C12-13 alkyl
  phosphate

potassium iodide

potassium myristate

PPG-30

propanediol

propyl gallate

propylene carbonate

propylene glycol

propylene glycol alginate

propylheptyl caprylate

propylparaben

providone
  (polyvinylpyrrolidone)

PVP/VA copolymer

quaternium-15

ricinoleylpropyl PG-dimonium
  chloride phosphate

salicylic acid

silica dimethyl silylate

silica silylate

silver citrate

simethicone

soapstone (talc)

sodium acrylate

sodium bisulfite

sodium C14-16 olefin
  sulfonate

sodium cetearyl sulfate

sodium coco-sulfate

sodium cocoyl sulfate

sodium erythorbate

sodium fluoride

sodium
  hydroxymethylglycinate

sodium isostearoyl lactylate

sodium laureth sulfate

sodium lauryl
  glucosideoxyacetate

sodium lauryl sulfate

sodium lauryl sulfoacetate

sodium methyl oleoyl taurate

sodium myreth sulfate

sodium PEG-7 olive oil
  carboxylate

sodium polyacrylate

sodium sulfate

sodium sulfite

sodium trideceth sulfate

sorbitan isostearate

soyamide DEA

soyamidopropalkonium
  chloride

squalane

stearamidopropyl dimethyl
  amine

steardimonium

steardimonium chloride

steareth-2, 20, 21, 100, etc.

stearoxytrimethylsilane

styrene-PVP copolymer

sulfated castor oil

synthetic fragrance

talc

tallow

TEA-carbomer

TEA-lauryl sulfate

tetrahexyldecyl ascorbate

tetrahydroxypropyl
  ethylenediamine

tetrasodium EDTA

thiotic acid

tin oxide

tri alkyl citrate

tribehenin

triclosan

tridecyl neopentanoate

tridecyl salicylate

triethanolamine (TEA)

triethoxycarpylysilane

trihydroxystearin

trimethylsiloxysilicate

trisodium EDTA (tetrasodium
  EDTA)

tromethamine stearate

tropolone

ultramarines

urea

vanillin

wheat germamidopropyl
  betaine

wheat germamidopropyl
  dimethylamine

zinc pyrithione

A BRIEF GUIDE TO BIOIDENTICAL HORMONE REPLACEMENT

Hormone replacement is an art, and it is crucial to find the right doctor, one who has chosen to specialize in bioidentical hormone replacement. Once you find yourself in the right office (go to SuzanneSomers.com for a doctor near you), then it is important you understand the different ways to take your hormones. I will explain both and you can make your own decision.

There are two correct ways to replace hormones: static dosing and rhythmic cycling. I have chosen to take my hormones in a natural rhythm, mimicking nature. But read the explanations below and decide for yourself. If you are menopausal and still have a uterus, you will be reactivating your monthly period. "What?" you ask. According to every doctor I have interviewed, it is crucial to replicate nature. Even though you may no longer have any or a sufficient number of eggs left, it is important for you to reset the hormonal clock. To do it any other way is to go against nature. Whenever we try to outthink nature we get in trouble. The argument that cessation of your menstrual period is natural is correct if you are choosing to age and not take advanatage of the advances in medicine. But think about it, every time you have an MRI or a CT scan, or take pharmaceutical drugs, even simple ones such as antibiotics, and utilize sewage treatment systems, you are prolonging life. Years ago people died early without the advantage of these new technologies. So to replace hormones that extend life and replicate your healthiest and optimal prime with good quality requires replacing hormones exactly the way nature once poured them into the body. In order to do this, having a monthly period is the only way to replicate nature and thereby be your healthiest and happiest self. Remember, you are choosing restoration versus deterioration.

"But still," you ask, "reactivate or perpetuate my period?" Yes, you are essentially tricking your body. The body knows that it produces estrogen every day of the month and for two weeks out of that month it produces progesterone. At the end of that cycle you get a period. It would confuse your body if you altered that pattern. When you confuse the body, you set yourself up to be sick and often very sick. So the way to be healthiest, happiest, and thinnest is to put the hormones back the way nature intended.

STATIC DOSING

With static dosing your doctor will most likely start you on low-dose bioidenticals according to your symptoms. After a couple of months he or she will order a blood test, approximate your hormone levels, and prescribe a static daily dose (constant amount) of estradiol and estriol. (Never, ever use estradiol without a greater quantity of estriol unless you know for sure that your body makes plenty of estriol on its own! Mine didn't, and that may be a big part of why I developed breast cancer!) On days 18 to 28, your doctor adds in a static dose of progesterone based upon your lab work. This regimen is designed to match what our bodies once made when we were making a full complement of hormones. It brings about a period at the end of each cycle at the end of the month.

So far it sounds simple, but here is the complex part.

Stress affects hormone production, so if you are going through a stressful period in your life it changes your needs. To compensate you may need to dose up or down a milligram. If the stress is severe you may need to have another blood test to determine where your levels are. This is the part I call an art form. It is important that you work closely with your doctor and communicate your symptoms (those seven dwarves) so he or she can adjust your dosages until they are just right.

If you are still making some hormones, meaning if your symptoms are mild but you are just not feeling "right," then static dosing seems to work quite well. As long as your body is still producing *some* hormones, as in women in their thirties, forties, and even early fifties, you are making your own rhythm and simply augmenting what is missing by replacing additional hormones with a static dose to re-create your optimal health.

Most doctors who have chosen to specialize in bioidentical hormones will prescribe hormones in this way. However there is another approach, it's called rhythmic cycling.

RHYTHMIC CYCLING

Rhythmic cycling is a new concept in bioidentical hormone replacement that is based upon the ancient cycles of nature. I take my hormones (including both estradiol and estriol) rhythmically, as prescribed by my doctor. At my age, my body is no longer making hormones, so I need complete replacement, and I also need to reestablish the rhythm of nature in my body for it to operate at its peak. I have found taking my hormones in a rhythm is best for me. Every woman is different, though, so use your own judgment as to which way most fits your needs.

The rhythm that this process refers to goes back to early man, who was attuned to the planet in a way that is completely inaccessible to us in the modern world. In ancient times women cycled to the rhythms of the moon. Our bodies would produce estrogen in increments: the first three days was one amount, the next three days another amount (each woman required the perfect amount for her) and by the twelfth day our estrogen would peak, which happened to coincide with the full moon. Then the receptor sites opened to receive progesterone, and the lining of the uterus would shed. As the estrogen fell, the progesterone would rise until it reached its incremental peak, only to rebuild the lining of the uterus to be ready the next month to start this process all over again. Our cycle of life.

Sound complicated? Not really.

Every month my syringes arrive in the mail along with a calendar indicating how much to take daily; the syringes have lines on them, each one representing a milligram. The calendar tells you how many milligrams to take on that particular day. It's really quite simple. I have been taking them for ten years in this way, and for me it is working great. I never have any symptoms and it is very easy to keep my weight under control. If you'd like more information about this method, visit www.suzanne somers.com.

Now you realize there are two ways to take prescribed bioidentical hormones and they both work. The choice is yours. If you are younger, perhaps static dosing will work best for you. If you are older than fifty, rhythmic cycling seems to work well. Either way, it's important to understand each individual hormone, what it does, and why it is important to your health, quality of life—and your waistline.

WHAT'S THE DIFFERENCE BETWEEN HRT AND BHRT?

Hormone replacement gets very confusing. So I'd like to clear up the differences between synthetic pharmaceutical hormones and synthetic pharmaceutical bioidentical hormones. Both of these are different from compounded, made-to-order, individualized bioidentical hormones. You need to know the difference when you get a prescription.

So many women write and tell me they are on BHRT (they think) and then mention names such as FemHRT and others. In putting this together, I asked Dr. Jonathan Wright to clear up the confusion:

> Precise definitions are tricky. Remember, bioidentical estrogens, progesterone, DHEA, tesosterone, are all *synthetic,* starting originally with material derived from yam or soy, but after chemical manipulation they end up finally as *bioidentical* to human hormones. That makes them the safest thing out there—when used properly!
>
> *Synthetic* means starting with one molecule, and altering it

through chemical processes into another molecule. The synthetic process is not good or bad in itself; it's the final molecule that is good or bad. For instance: Premarin is not synthetic, it's totally natural—to a horse—but *not at all bioidentical* for humans. That's why it's dangerous.

Here is a list describing a number of different available hormones:

Premarin: Natural horse estrogens; not bioidentical to human estrogen

Provera: Synthetic not bioidentical

Prochieve, Crinon: Synthetic but bioidentical to human progesterone; difficult to individualize

Synapause-E3: Synthetic and bioidentical, but taken orally, so it is not safe. Oral estrogens, even bioidentical, raise risk. BHRT should always be transdermal or transmucosal.

Cenestin, Enjuvia: Synthetic horse estrogens (Natural horse estrogens are bad enough; why synthesize 'em?)

FemHRT: Synthetic estrogens (like those usually found in birth control pills)

Bioidentical Hormones Safely Used in BHRT

Estradiol: Synthetic but bioidentical—used in BHRT in combination with estriol

Estriol: Synthetic but bioidentical—used in BHRT in combination with estradiol

Progesterone: Synthetic but bioidentical

DHEA: Synthetic but bioidentical

Testosterone: Synthetic but bioidentical

RESOURCES

The doctors and professionals in this list are experts in their chosen fields. I have personally worked with some of them; others have been referred from trusted sources. That being said, I cannot guarantee your satisfaction with any of these professionals. Please use this list as a starting point, then interview each doctor to see who fits your particular needs. I always appreciate your feedback.

For a complete list of integrative health care practitioners providing support for BHRT, optimal health, antiaging, and healing from various disease conditions, as well as a list of compounding pharmacies and Ondamed practitioners, please go to SuzanneSomers.com where they are listed by state and country.

SEXY FOREVER PLAN

Sexy Forever's online companion, available at SexyForever.com/book, includes tools and support that will make finding lifelong health and slimness so easy. You'll receive a customized daily meal planner to guide you through each step of my plan, plus have access to hundreds of delicious recipes, personal weight and inch trackers, an online journal to help track your progress, and printable wallet-sized shopping lists and food guides to keep in your purse or take with you on the go. When you join SexyForever.com/book, you'll become a member of a supportive community of like-minded people with similar health goals, who share advice and words of encouragement in the message board forums. You'll even be able to enlist one-on-one support from a Sexy Forever nutrition coach. And of course I'll be there every step of the way: You'll receive a daily Sexy Forever newsletter with plenty of motivational advice from me, plus healthy eating and detoxification tips, news, updates, and everything you'll need to stay Sexy Forever. Visit SexyForever.com/book.

BLOOD TESTS THAT UNCOVER HIDDEN FACTORS OF WEIGHT GAIN

An analysis of your blood can uncover biological abnormalities that may be causing or contributing to unwanted weight gain. Appropriate blood tests can also reveal silent conditions that predispose you to increased risks of cancer, heart attack, stroke, and dementia.

Once you receive your blood test results, you possess the knowledge to *reverse* undesirable factors that are an underlying cause of a variety of health maladies, including surplus fat accumulation.

Here are some obesity-inducing factors that are included in the Comprehensive Weight Loss Blood Test Panel.

1. **Estradiol (a type of estrogen).** Suboptimal levels of estrogen are associated with weight gain in women, especially in the abdominal area. Several studies show a *reduction* in abdominal obesity in women in response to restoration of estrogen balance. In fact, many experts in the field of bioidentical hormone replacement therapy report impressive improvements in body composition in peri- and post-menopausal women once hormone balance is restored. If a woman's blood test shows estrogen levels are low, she can be prescribed bioidentical estrogen to restore it to a more youthful level.

   In men, low testosterone in combination with *excess* estrogen is associated with excess abdominal fat mass. There are several methods to restore optimal hormone balance (including estrogen) in men. That is why estradiol levels are included in the male and female Weight Loss Blood Test Panels.

Experts in bioidentical hormone replacement therapy strive to achieve optimal results by working in harmony with each individual's unique biochemistry, carefully titrating bioidentical hormone dosages with blood levels as well as biological effects. For menopausal and postmenopausal women, most experts in bioidentical hormone replacement therapy believe the optimal *estradiol* blood level range is 90 to 250 pg/mL. For men, most experts believe the optimal estradiol range is 20 to 30 pg/mL.

In addition, bioidentical hormone replacement experts believe that it is important for women to keep their *progesterone* blood level between 2.0 and 6.0 pg/mL, especially if they are taking supplemental estrogen (preferably in bioidentical forms discussed in this book).

2. **Testosterone.** Low levels of testosterone in men are associated with visceral adiposity (i.e., fat that surrounds the organs of the abdominal cavity). When men deficient in testosterone are given supplementary bioidentical testosterone, the result is often a *decrease* in belly fat. In postmenopausal women, relatively low estrogen and higher-than-optimal testosterone can contribute to an *increase* in abdominal fat mass. Furthermore, some young women with excess body fat suffer from an underlying medical condition characterized by elevated testosterone, insulin resistance, and menstrual irregularities. Many people do not know that this medical problem, called polycystic ovary syndrome (PCOS), is one of the most common hormone abnormalities that occur in women of reproductive age. There are several ways to restore balance between estrogen and testosterone in women. That is why testosterone levels are included in the male and female Weight Loss Blood Test Panels.

Many experts in testosterone restoration therapy believe that men (who do not have prostate cancer) should maintain their *free testosterone* in the range of 20 to 25 pg/mL, which is approximately the upper third range for free testosterone observed in young men, whereas women should keep their free testosterone blood level much lower, at 1.0 to 2.2 pg/mL.

3. **Thyroid.** The rate of cellular energy expenditure is regulated partially by T3 thyroid hormone. Low thyroid predisposes women and men to weight gain. The Weight Loss Blood Test Panel checks free T3, free T4, and thyroid stimulating hormone (TSH). If deficient, thyroid hormone replacement can be prescribed. Optimal free T3 and free T4 levels are at the upper one-third range of normal. The normal range for *TSH* is typically between 0.3 and 3.0 mIU/mL, but for optimal thyroid status, a TSH of greater than 2.0 mIU/mL may predispose one to weight gain. When TSH is elevated, this suggests reduced thyroid hormone output as the body's endocrine system tries to compensate by secreting more thyroid stimulating hormone (TSH).

4. **Triglycerides.** This test is used to identify coronary heart disease risk, but it can also uncover fat metabolism disorders. An elevated fasting triglyceride level has been identified as an independent risk factor for vascular disease. However, many people do not realize that in the context of weight loss, experimental studies indicate that higher than optimal levels of triglycerides after eating (such as 2 to 4 hours following a meal) can predict the risk of diet-induced obesity. Clinical studies suggest that the optimal level for *non-fasting triglycerides* (the level of triglycerides 2 to 4 hours following a meal) is no more than 116 mg/dL, above which there is an increase in risk of heart disease and stroke. There are a number of proven methods to reduce excess triglycerides from your bloodstream that may better enable you to reduce your risk. Optimal *fasting triglyceride* levels to strive for are 80 mg/dL or less.

5. **Glucose.** Excess blood sugar induces metabolic havoc and is often associated with excess body weight, in particular excess visceral fat. Many people are not aware that a number of studies suggest that chronic elevations in insulin and blood sugar can impair the brain's appetite regulating mechanism. Even when fasting blood sugar levels are in the upper normal ranges, you may still suffer from impaired glucose tolerance associated with insulin resistance. Insulin resistance

causes your pancreas to pump out more insulin in the attempt to drive nutrients into cells. However, burning body fat is difficult in the presence of elevated levels of insulin. Glucose elevation is also associated with activation of genes that induce body fat formation. Fortunately there are several proven methods to safely restore glucose levels to an optimal level. An optimal *fasting glucose* range to strive for is 70 to 85 mg/dL.

6. **C-reactive protein.** Excess C-reactive protein interferes with the ability of leptin to control appetite and burn fat. If your C-reactive protein levels are elevated, it is important to follow the steps discussed in this book to suppress this marker of chronic inflammation (C-reactive protein) in your body. A side benefit to lowering C-reactive protein is a reduction in the risk of heart attack and stroke. Men should have a *C-reactive protein* blood level of 0.55 mg/L or less, while women should have 1.50 mg/L or less of C-reactive protein.

7. **Food sensitivities.** Many people don't realize that various forms of food sensitivity can create a chronic low level of inflammation that can disable some of the body's fat storage regulatory mechanisms. Reactions to food can also be a hidden cause behind an array of health problems, including headaches and migraines, insomnia, and digestive disorders. An advanced, convenient diagnostic blood test technology called the FoodSafe test enables you and your doctor to zero in on the potential foods behind your health problems and methodically eliminate them.

8. **Omega-3 Score.** Based on an overwhelming volume of published documentation, health-conscious Americans are gulping down fish oil and other supplements that provide essential omega-3 fatty acids. What a lot of people don't realize is that dosing of omega-3s varies considerably among individuals. Many people who think they are getting enough EPA/DHA omega-3s are not. A new at-home Omega-3 Score blood test measures your individual fatty acid status so you can

optimize your body's omega-3 to omega-6 balance. Research suggests that relatively deficient levels of omega-3 in the presence of excess omega-6 can contribute to systemic inflammation in the body, insulin resistance, and difficulty with weight management.

9. **Heavy Metals Profile.** Even those who try to eat healthfully can inadvertently suffer buildup of heavy metals such as mercury, lead, and arsenic. This is becoming a problem as more people eat seafood that has been contaminated with industrial pollutants. Blood or urine tests can reveal if you need to remove (chelate) these heavy metals from your body.

10. *H. pylori.* A strikingly high percentage of the population is infected with the *Helicobacter pylori* bacteria. This bacterium resides in the stomach and can create serious health issues, including stomach cancer, if not eradicated. An *H. pylori* antibody blood test can help detect this insidious bacteria and enable you to take steps to eliminate it from your body.

11. **Vitamin D.** Overweight and obese individuals are often vitamin D deficient. The problem with insufficient vitamin D is that this is often accompanied by systemic inflammation that can sabotage the best weight loss plans. Remember that pro-inflammatory compounds like C-reactive protein can bind to leptin and deactivate leptin's natural antiobesity effects. Most people need to take at least 5,000 IU a day of supplemental vitamin D to achieve vitamin D blood levels (measured as 25-hydroxy vitamin D) of at least 50 ng/mL. Many aging individuals who avoid sun exposure out of concern for skin cancer and skin aging require 5,000 to 8,000 IU of vitamin D_3 daily to achieve optimal levels in the body. A blood test for 25-hydroxy vitamin D should be obtained within two months of vitamin D_3 supplementation to ascertain the body's response.

HOW TO OBTAIN THESE BLOOD TESTS AT AFFORDABLE PRICES

Comprehensive blood tests from commercial laboratories can be quite costly, but I have arranged for my readers to obtain special low prices for them. The good news is that you can order these tests yourself and have your blood drawn in a blood drawing station near you at your convenience.

At a minimum, anyone seeking to lose weight should obtain a Comprehensive Weight Loss Blood Test Panel that includes C-reactive protein, estradiol, thyroid, testosterone, glucose, triglycerides, progesterone (for women), PSA (for men), and numerous other health markers. You can order this comprehensive blood test today by logging on to Suzanne Somers.com and clicking on Life Extension or calling 1-888-884-3666.

When you get your test results back, Life Extension maintains a dedicated team of health advisers that can assist in using your individual blood tests to facilitate healthy weight loss. These health advisers are available seven days a week and can be reached by calling 1-888-884-3666.

THE LIFE EXTENSION FOUNDATION

The Life Extension Foundation is the largest antiaging medicine organization in the world. Since 1980, this nonprofit group has uncovered validated methods to slow premature aging and treat degenerative disease.

My readers can obtain a free copy of the most current issue of *Life Extension* magazine by calling 1-888-884-3625 or logging on to SuzanneSomers .com and clicking on Life Extension.

I receive *Life Extension* magazine each month and stop whatever I am doing to read it cover to cover. I do this because Life Extension has a track record of introducing evidence-based approaches to enhancing longevity that are five to ten years ahead of conventional medicine. These life-saving scientific advances are chronicled each month in *Life Extension* magazine, read by more than 400,000 people worldwide.

Consumers and medical professionals alike read *Life Extension* magazine to obtain the latest information about achieving long life, while protecting against common age-related disorders such as obesity.

NEW TECHNOLOGIES

All three of these companies can be contacted by direct links on my website, SuzanneSomers.com.

David Schmidt
LifeWave
1020 Prospect St., Suite 200
La Jolla, CA 92037
858-459-9876
866-420-6288
SuzanneSomers.com (click on LifeWave)

Robin Smith, MD, MBA
NeoStem, Inc.
420 Lexington Ave., Suite 450
New York, NY 10170
212-584-4180
646-514-7787 (fax)
SuzanneSomers.com (click on NeoStem)

Ondamed
SuzanneSomers.com (click on Ondamed)

FOOD INTOLERANCE TEST

Dr. Kenneth Fine
(best known for isolating antibodies for gluten in the stool)
Enterolab
10986 Plano Rd.
Dallas, TX 75238
972-686-6869
www.enterolab.com

Meridian Valley Lab
425-271-8689
www.MeridianValleyLab.com
Meridian Valley Lab can help you identify your food allergies, including hidden food sensitivities. By testing for antibodies of up to 190 foods, you get a good idea of foods you may want to avoid. You can begin your test at home with a simple finger-prick kit called the Food Safe Allergy Test or have your blood drawn at a lab for their E-95, A-95, or E-95/A-95 Combo panel for a reduced price. When you get your food allergy report, you'll also receive a food rotation diet guide that will help you get started on a better road to health and wellness. Of course, any weight loss is free of charge!

OTHER HELPFUL WEBSITES

Dr. Russell L. Blaylock
Advanced Nutritional Concepts, LLC
www.russellblaylockmd.com
www.newportnutritionals.com
Blaylock Wellness Report: www.blaylockreport.com

Julie Carmen
www.JulieCarmenYoga.com
www.yogatalks.com

Designs for Health
www.designsforhealth.com

Don Tolman
www.dontolmaninternational.com

Brenda Watson
www.renewlife.com

TESTING HORMONE LEVELS

Aeron LifeCycles
1933 Davis St., Suite 310
San Leandro, CA 94577
800-631-7900
www.aeron.com

Life Extension Foundation
Fort Lauderdale, FL
888-884-3666
www.lef.org/goodhealth

Sabre Sciences, Inc.
2233 Faraday Ave., Suite K
Carlsbad, CA 92008
www.sabresciences.com

TESTING FOR NUTRITIONAL DEFICIENCIES

Doctor's Data
3755 Illinois Ave.
St. Charles, IL 60174-2420
800-323-2784 (USA, Canada)
0871-218-0052 (United Kingdom)
Email: inquiries@doctorsdata.com
www.doctorsdata.com

Genova Diagnostics
63 Zillicoa St.
Asheville, NC 28801
800-522-4762
www.gdx.net

Metametrix Clinical Laboratories
4855 Peachtree Industrial Blvd.
Norcross, GA 30092
770-446-5483
www.metametrix.com

Cristiana Paul, MS
Los Angeles, CA
Email: cristiana@cristianapaul.com
www.cristianapaul.com

SUZANNE ORGANICS BEAUTY PRODUCTS

SuzanneSomers.com (click on Beauty)

RESTORE LIFE FORMULAS VITAMINS AND SUPPLEMENTS

SuzanneSomers.com (click on Supplements)

PERSONAL CARE

SomerSmile Get White Tooth Whitening System
LifeWave Nanotechnology patches
Life Extension for blood testing
NeoStem for stem cell collection information
FaceMaster
Visit SuzanneSomers.com for more information on each.

EXERCISE PRODUCTS

ThighMaster
www.thighmaster.com

EZ Gym
www.ezgym.com

Torso Track
SuzanneSomers.com

ORGANIC FIBER

www.renewlife.com

Organic Clear Fiber is soluble and helps with managing cholesterol, soaking up toxins in the gut, and weight loss.

FiberSmart is flax with soluble and insoluble plus soothing herbs. Good for a fiber supplement, but also great for IBS.

Organic Triple Fiber has both soluble and insoluble. It is a general overall good fiber supplement.

Fibertastic is 50 percent soluble and 50 percent insoluble. The benefit of this fiber is it tastes so good even kids will eat it in their diets. It is made from fruit and vegetable fiber and it smells like pears.

RECOMMENDED READING

Amsterdam, Elana (www.elanaspantry.com). *The Gluten-Free Almond Flour Cookbook.* Berkeley, Calif.: Celestial Arts, 2009.

Begley, Ed, Jr. (www.edbegley.com). *Ed Begley, Jr.'s Guide to Sustainable Living.* New York: Clarkson Potter, 2009.

———. *Living Like Ed.* New York: Clarkson Potter, 2008.

Begley, Ed, Jr., Rick McLean, and Dr. David Suzuki. *Grassroots Rising.* Kansas City: Honour Group Publishing, 2006.

Blaylock, Russell L., M.D. (www.russellblaylockmd.com). *Excitotoxins: The Taste That Kills.* Royal Oak, Mich.: Health Press, 1996.

———. *Health and Nutrition Secrets That Can Save Your Life,* revised edition. Royal Oak, Mich.: Health Press, 2006.

———. *Natural Strategies for Cancer Patients.* London: Kensington, 2003.

———. *Nuclear Sunrise* (e-booklet).

Braverman, Eric R., M.D. (www.pathmed.com). *The Edge Effect: Achieve Total Health and Longevity with the Balanced Brain Advantage.* New York: Sterling, 2005.

———. *Younger You: Unlock the Hidden Power of Your Brain to Look and Feel 15 Years Younger.* New York: McGraw-Hill, 2008.

Brownlee, Shannon (www.overtreated.com). *Overtreated: Why Too Much Medicine Is Making Us Sicker and Poorer.* New York: Bloomsbury, 2008.

The Burton Goldberg Group (www.burtongoldberg.com). *Alternative Medicine: The Definitive Guide.* London: Future Medicine Publishing, 1995.

Canton, James M., Ph.D. (www.globalfuturist.com). *The Extreme Future: The Top Trends That Will Reshape the World for the Next 5, 10, and 20 Years.* New York: Dutton, 2006.

Carson, Rachel. *Silent Spring.* New York: Mariner, 2002.

Colgan, Dr. Michael. *Hormonal Health*. Vancouver: Apple Publishing, 1996.

Crinnion, Walter, N.D. (www.crinnionmedical.com). *Clean, Green, and Lean*. New York: Wiley, 2010.

Fallon, Sally (www.sallyfallon.com). *Nourishing Traditions*. Lanham, Md.: NewTrends Publishing, 1999.

Gonzalez, Nicholas, M.D. (www.dr-gonzalez.com). *One Man Alone*. New York: New Spring Press, 2010.

Graveline, Duane, M.D. *Lipitor: Thief of Memory*. Self-published, 2006.

Greene, Robert A., M.D. (www.robertgreenemd.com), and Leah Feldon. *Perfect Balance: Dr. Robert Greene's Breakthrough Program for Finding the Lifelong Hormonal Health You Deserve*. New York: Clarkson Potter, 2005.

Hertoghe, Thierry, M.D. (www.hertoghe.eu). *The Hormone Solution*. New York: Three Rivers Press, 2002.

Kurzweil, Ray (www.kurzweilai.net), and Terry Grossman, M.D. *Fantastic Voyage*. New York: Plume, 2005.

Lieberman, Shari, Ph.D., CNS, FACN. *The Gluten Connection*. Emmaus, Pa.: Rodale, 2006.

Life Extension Foundation (www.lef.org). *Disease Prevention and Treatment*, expanded fourth edition. Fort Lauderdale, Fla.: Life Extension, 2003.

———. *FDA Failure, Deception, Abuse*. Edinburg, Va.: Praktikos Books, 2010.

Mahmud, Khalid, M.D. (www.idinhealth.com). *Keeping aBreast: Ways to Stop Breast Cancer*. Bloomington, Ind.: AuthorHouse, 2005.

Martino, Russell J., Ph.D. (www.drrussellshealthandweightlossblog.com). *5 Steps to Optimal Health*.

Mercola, Joseph (www.mercola.com). *Take Control of Your Health* (2007).

Miller, Philip Lee, M.D. (www.antiaging.com), and the Life Extension Foundation (www.lef.org). *Life Extension Revolution: The New Science of Growing Older Without Aging*. New York: Bantam, 2006.

Murphy, Christine, ed. *Iscador: Mistletoe and Cancer Therapy*. Herndon, Va.: Lantern Books, 2001.

Niehans, Paul. *Introduction to Cellular Therapy.* New York: Pageant Books, 1960.

Pizzorno, Joseph E., and Michael T. Murray, eds. *The Textbook of Natural Medicine,* third edition. St. Louis, Mo.: Churchill Livingstone, 2006.

Ragnar, Peter (www.peterragnar.com). *The Lifewave Experience to a New You! The Official Handbook.* Asheville, N.C.: Roaring Lion Publishing, 2007.

Rogers, Sherry A., M.D. (www.healthywealthyandwise.com). *Detoxify or Die.* Hampton, Va.: Prestige, 2002.

Rothenberg, Ron, M.D. (www.ehealthspan.com), Kathleen Becker, and Kris Hart. *Forever Ageless, Advanced Edition.* Encinitas, Calif.: Health-Span Institute, 2007.

Simpson, Kathryn R., M.S. (www.themssolution.com). *The Women's Guide to Thyroid Health.* Oakland, Calif.: New Harbinger, 2009.

Small, Gary, M.D., with Gigi Vorgan. *The Longevity Bible.* New York: Hyperion, 2007.

Somers, Suzanne (www.SuzanneSomers.com). *Ageless.* New York: Three Rivers Press, 2007.

———. *Breakthrough.* New York: Three Rivers Press, 2009.

———. *The Sexy Years.* New York: Three Rivers Press, 2005.

———. *Slim and Sexy Forever.* New York: Three Rivers Press, 2006.

Starr, Mark, M.D. (www.21centurymed.com). *Hypothyroidism Type 2.* Irvine, Calif.: New Voice Publications, 2005.

Thomas, John. *Young Again: How to Reverse the Aging Process.* Medford, N.J.: Plexus Press, 2002.

Turner, Natasha, N.D. (www.clearmedicine.com). *The Hormone Diet.* Emmaus, Pa.: Rodale, 2010.

Van Zyl, Bernard. *Stem Cells Saved My Life: How to Be Next.* Bloomington, Ind.: AuthorHouse, 2006.

Virgin, J. J. (www.jjvirgin.com). *Six Weeks to Sleeveless and Sexy.* New York: Gallery, 2010.

Watson, Brenda, M.D. (www.renewlife.com). *The Detox Strategy.* New York: Free Press, 2008.

———. *The Fiber 35 Diet.* New York: Free Press, 2008.

————. *The HOPE Formula*. Palm Harbor, Fla.: ReNew Life Press, 2007.

Watson, Brenda, M.D., and Leonard Smith, M.D. *Gut Solutions: Natural Solutions to Your Digestive Problems*. Palm Harbor, Fla.: ReNew Life Press, 2004.

Wright, Jonathan V., M.D. (www.tahomaclinic.com). *Dr. Wright's Book of Nutritional Therapy: Real Life Lessons in Medicine Without Drugs*. Emmaus, Pa.: Rodale, 1979.

————. *Maximize Your Vitality and Potency*. Petaluma, Calif.: Smart Publications, 1999.

Wright, Jonathan V., M.D., et al. *The Natural Pharmacy*. New York: Three Rivers Press, 1999.

Wright, Jonathan V., M.D., and Alan R. Gaby, M.D. *Natural Medicine, Optimal Wellness* (formerly *Patient's Book of Natural Healing*). Ridgefield, Conn.: Vital Health Publishing, 2006.

Wright, Jonathan V., M.D., and Lane Lenard. *D-Mannose and Bladder Infection: The Natural Alternative to Antibiotics*. Auburn, Wash.: Dragon Art, 2001.

————. *Why Stomach Acid Is Good for You*. New York: M. Evans and Company, 2001.

————. *Xylitol: Dental and Upper Respiratory Health*. Auburn, Wash.: Dragon Art, 2003.

Wright, Jonathan V., M.D., and John Morgenthaler. *Natural Hormone Replacement for Women Over 45*. Petaluma, Calif.: Smart Publications, 1997.

Wright, Jonathan V., M.D., and John Neustadt. *Thriving Through Dialysis*. Auburn, Wash.: Dragon Art, 2005.

Young, Simon. *Designer Evolution: A Transhumanist Manifesto*. Amherst, N.Y.: Prometheus, 2005.

INDEX

RECIPE INDEX

Also by Suzanne Somers

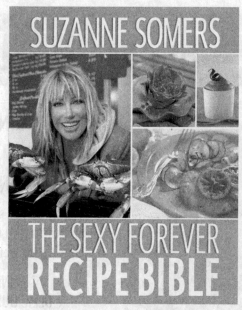

The Sexy Forever Recipe Bible
$21.99 Paperback (Canada: $24.99)
978-0-307-95670-5

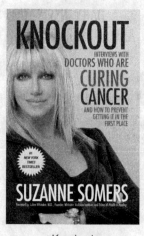

Knockout
Interviews with Doctors Who Are Curing Cancer
—And How to Prevent Getting It in the First Place
$15.00 Paperback (Canada: $17.00)
978-0-307-58759-6

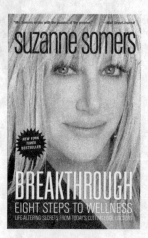

Breakthrough
Eight Steps to Wellness
$15.00 Paperback (Canada: $18.95)
978-1-4000-5328-5

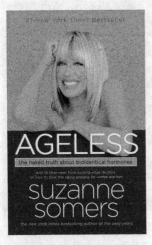

Ageless
The Naked Truth About Bioidentical Hormones
$15.00 Paperback (Canada: $18.95)
978-0-307-23725-5

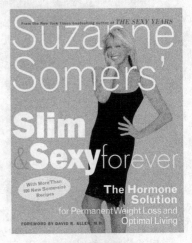

Slim and Sexy Forever
The Hormone Solution for Permanent Weight Loss
and Optimal Living
$17.99 Paperback (Canada: $22.99)
978-1-4000-5326-1

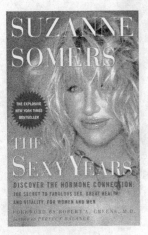

The Sexy Years
Discover the Hormone Connection: The
Secret to Fabulous Sex, Great Health, and
Vitality, for Women and Men
$15.00 Paperback (Canada: $18.95)
978-1-4000-8157-8

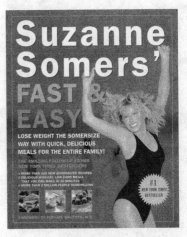

Fast & Easy
Lose Weight the Somersize Way with Quick,
Delicious Meals for the Entire Family!
$16.95 Paperback (Canada: $18.95)
978-1-4000-5296-7

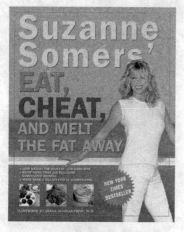

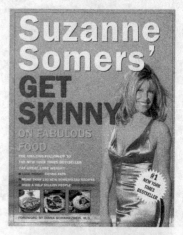

Eat, Cheat, and Melt the Fat Away
$18.99 Paperback (Canada: $20.99)
978-1-4000-4706-2

Get Skinny on Fabulous Food
$17.99 Paperback (Canada: $22.99)
978-0-609-80237-3

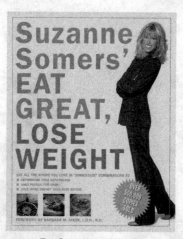

Eat Great, Lose Weight
$17.95 Paperback (Canada: $21.00)
978-0-609-80058-4

Available wherever books are sold.

THREE RIVERS PRESS · NEW YORK